I Dance for
Physical Literacy
12 Steps

Healthy Lifestyle Changes, Inc
501 (c) 3
New York, N.Y.
Visit:Physicalliteracy12steps.com
Copyright (c) 2015
All Rights Reserved

i

Physical Literacy
12 Steps Pledge
Ambassadorship

Library of Congress Control Number: 2015900286
Healthy Lifestyle Changes, Incorporated, Far Rockaway, 11691

THE WAVE, ROCKAWAY BEACH, N.Y., FRIDAY, NOVEMBER 22, 2013 - Page 86

Rockaway Walks Fitness Column
The Greatest Blessing

By Steven C. McCartney
IPO, HSW MS

It has been a blessing writing for The Wave newspaper and guiding you with important science-based evidence and information on staying mentally, physically and socially fit. Occasionally, I have reflected on past experiences to help you understand my philosophy towards being healthy. Even so, nothing can prepare you for what you are about to read. This article is about a special relationship between two individuals who have a child together, and are able to reunite after some time apart. In writing this article, my goal is to inspire individuals young and old to build strong relationships.

I met Tracey, the mother of Andre, 33 years ago on a college campus on Long Island, New York. Our families only accepted our relationship as far as we could see, which really wasn't all that far, since we were only about 18 at that time. We were lovers who were intimate, young and foolish, and this combination is a recipe for failure.

Within three years after beginning our relationship, Tracey became pregnant with our son, Andre. Personally I was not ready for fatherhood. I had not had the opportunity to live on my own, and I had just recently started to work for a utility company on Long Island. I was also not ready to meet the needs of the relationship between Tracey and me. Tracey was very hurt by the things that were going on and soon after Andre was born she left to join the military.

By the time Andre was two years of age, Tracey had other relationships and other children. To her credit, she raised the children as a single parent while in

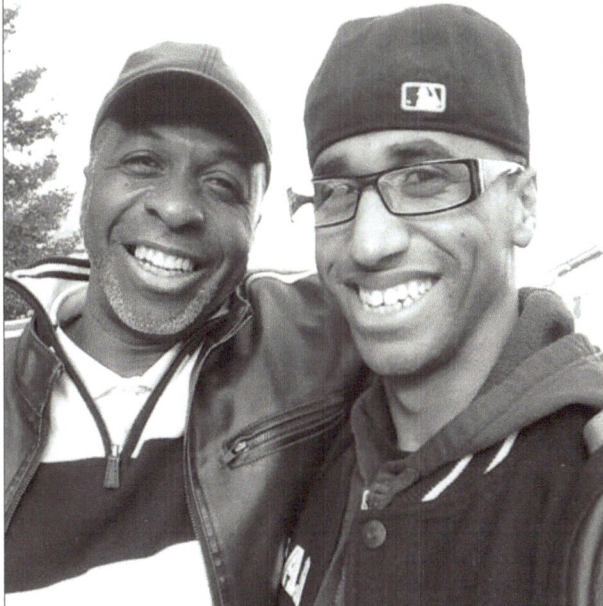

the armed services and has since retired from the federal government.

Over the years, my life has continued to take a number of twists and turns. I was emotionally hurt, and never recovered from the lack of resources to form a support team (review The Wave *Article FORM A SUPPORT TEAM*). I always wanted to know about Andre, my only son, but lacked information on Tracey's whereabouts until very recently.

Tracey started a Facebook account in 2013, and she requested me as a friend. This was my golden opportunity to be reunited with her, but I was also feeling many emotions. Some of these emotions were good, while others were not so positive. In the beginning, the conversation between the two of us was cordial, but it later became awkward, as tough questions began to be asked and emotions and concerns were also expressed.

A little while later, Tracey provided me with a contact number. In August 2013, we spoke for the first time in about 27 years. It was then that we first started to listen to each other and articulate our feelings and emotions. Tracey sent me a surprise e-mail with a series of photos that Andre had given her. Tracey talked so proudly of Andre's professional work as dance instructor and choreographer in ballroom, Latin, and Hip-hop dancing.

I was blown away, and if you have been following my work with Rockaway Walks, you know I am a veteran, writer for The Wave newspaper and a NYS Certified Physical Education Teacher, Swim Coach, and Founder of Healthy Lifestyle Changes, Inc. (501 c 3).

The growth of our relationship led Tracey and me to schedule a routine that required talking daily. The result of our conversations and the photos motivated us to start a project, a children's book called *The Dancer: Physical Literacy* using Andre's dance photos. Tracey finally notified her family that I was the father of Andre prior to me traveling to the West Coast to be by her side. After

that, I spoke to Andre for the first time over the phone. Tracey and I signed the book "From father and mother, love always", and mailed it overnight to Andre. Upon my return to the East Coast, Andre reached out to me in excitement. In October, 2013, Andre and I reunited (see photo) for the first time in 30 years. I am overjoyed.

Today, Tracey, Andre and I continue to communicate daily, and are working to build our lives together. I believe there are many individuals with families that have similar stories and I am so happy to be able to share with you one of my greatest blessings and happiest moments of my life. Tracey and Andre, I Love You.

This article goes out to the community of Rockaway Walks and Sponsors: Councilman Donovan Richards, St. John's Episcopal Hospital, Joseph Addabbo Health Center, Modell's Sporting Goods, Stop N Shop, NYC Parks & Recreation, York College, Healthy Lifestyle Changes Inc., VESID and The Wave newspaper. For Questions or comments contact Steven_mccartney @walkprograms.com

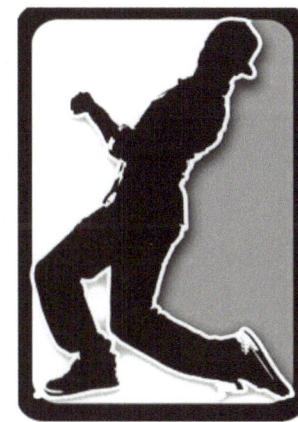

I Dance for *Physical Literacy* 12 Steps

Table of Content

iii

Introduction

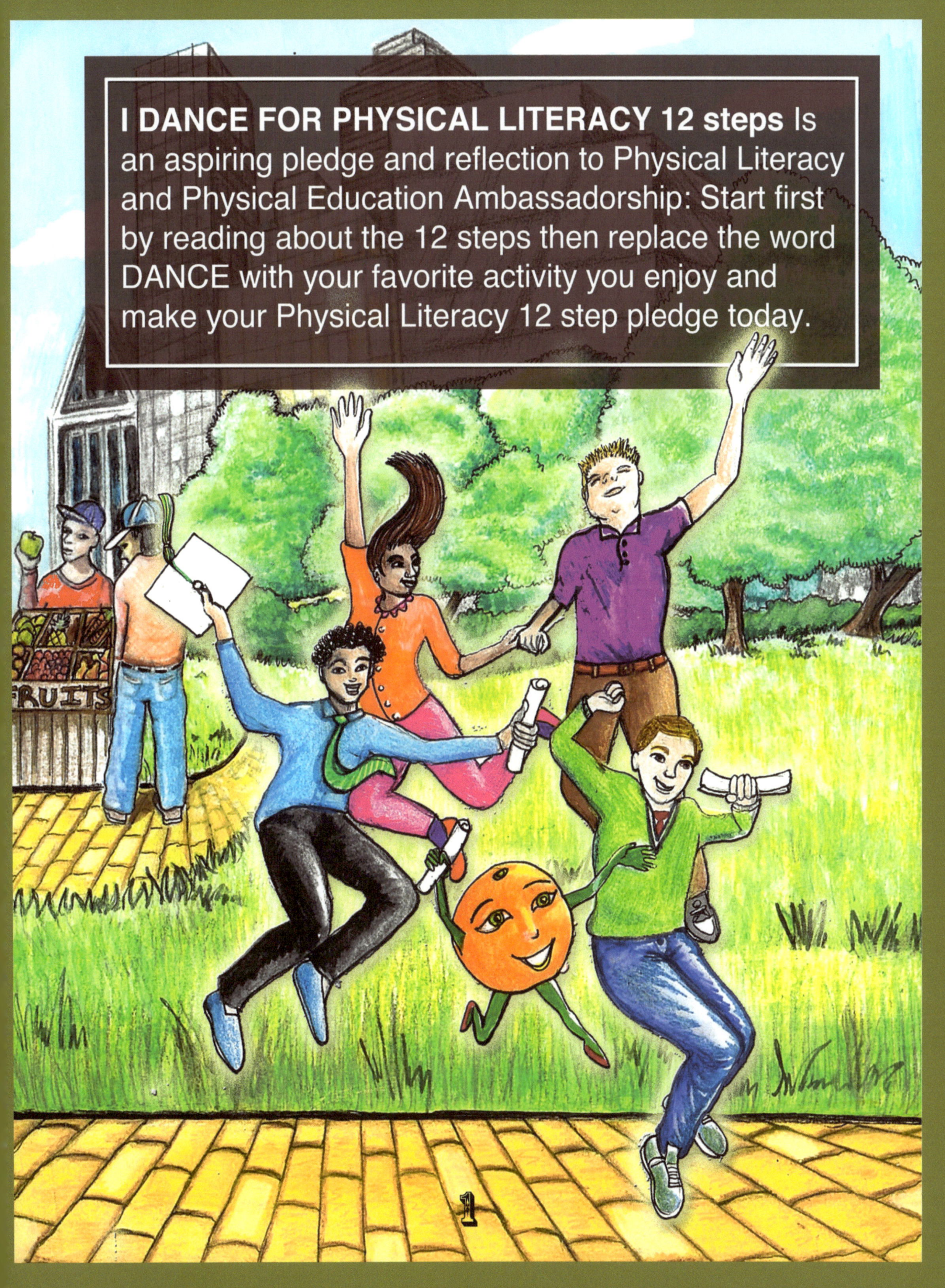

I DANCE FOR PHYSICAL LITERACY 12 steps Is an aspiring pledge and reflection to Physical Literacy and Physical Education Ambassadorship: Start first by reading about the 12 steps then replace the word DANCE with your favorite activity you enjoy and make your Physical Literacy 12 step pledge today.

Physical Literacy
1st
Step

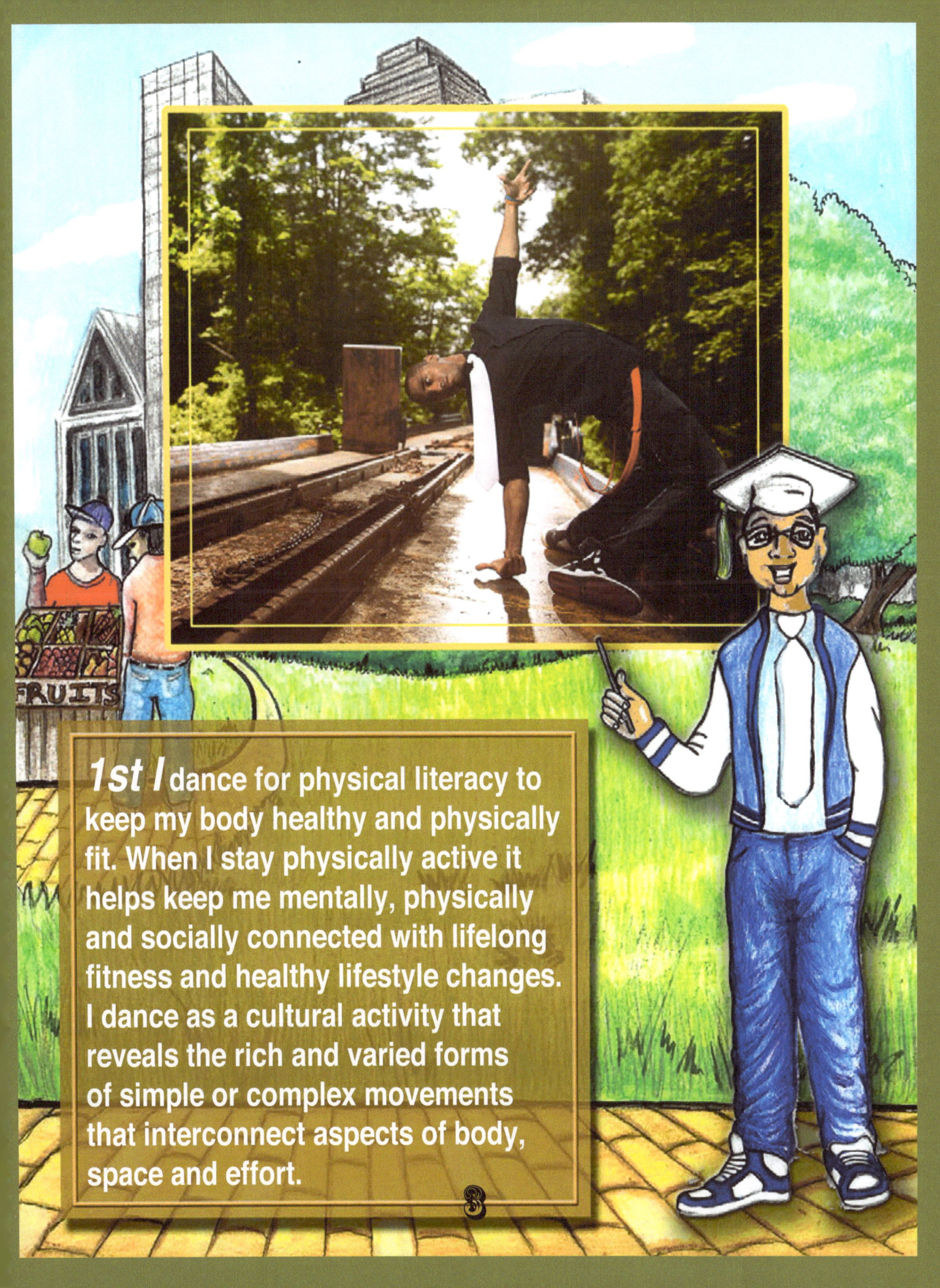

1st I dance for physical literacy to keep my body healthy and physically fit. When I stay physically active it helps keep me mentally, physically and socially connected with lifelong fitness and healthy lifestyle changes. I dance as a cultural activity that reveals the rich and varied forms of simple or complex movements that interconnect aspects of body, space and effort.

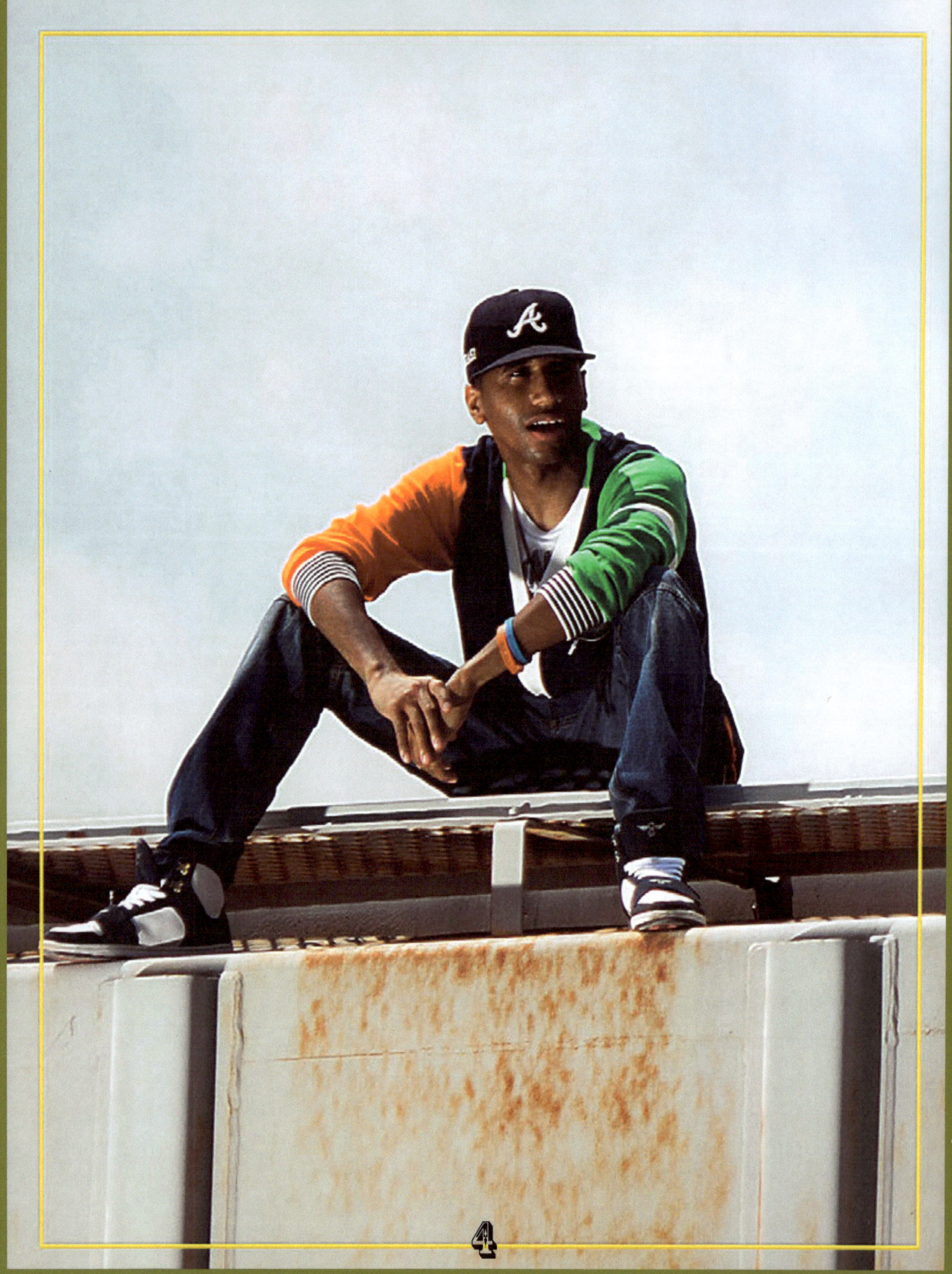

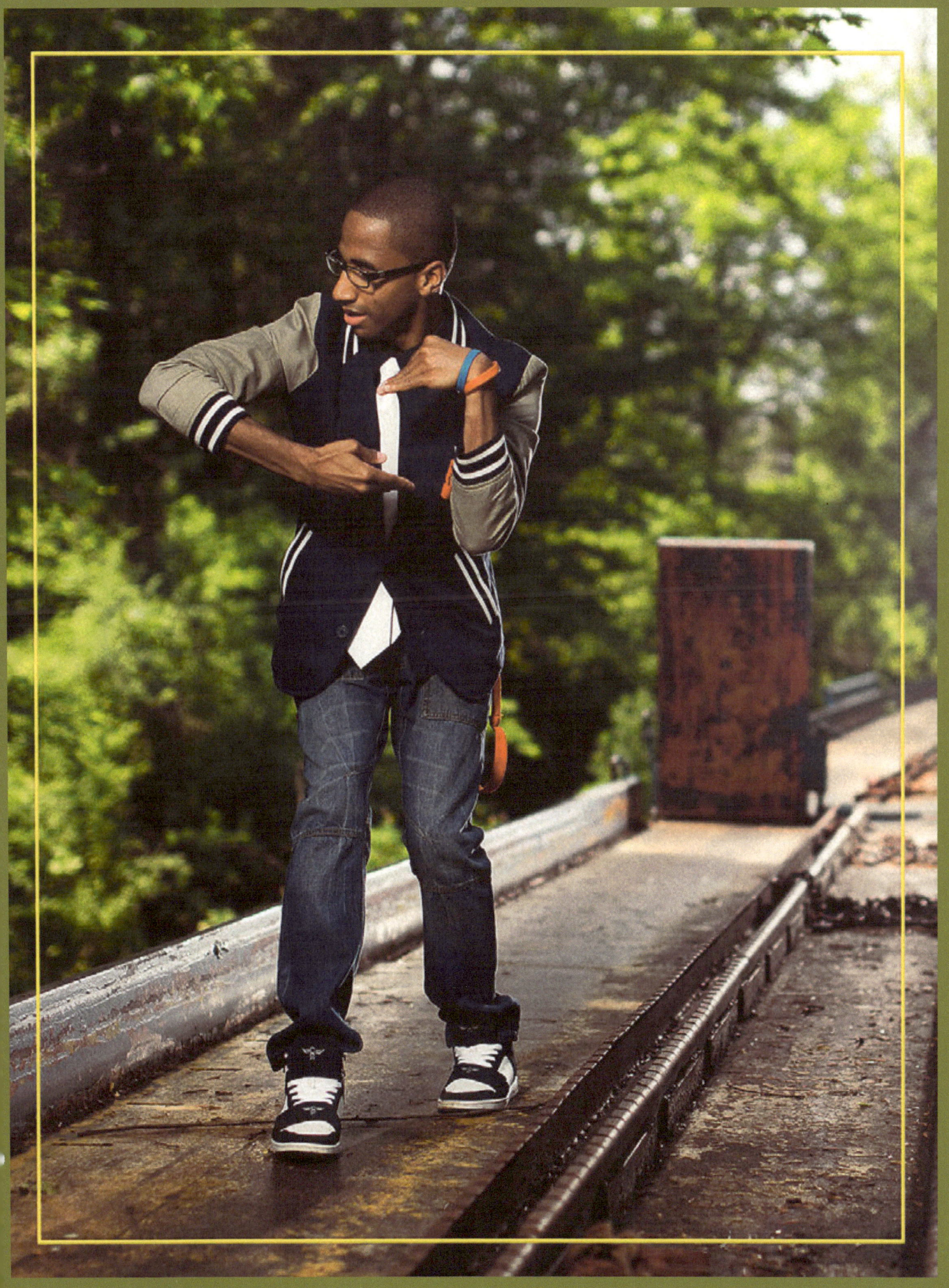

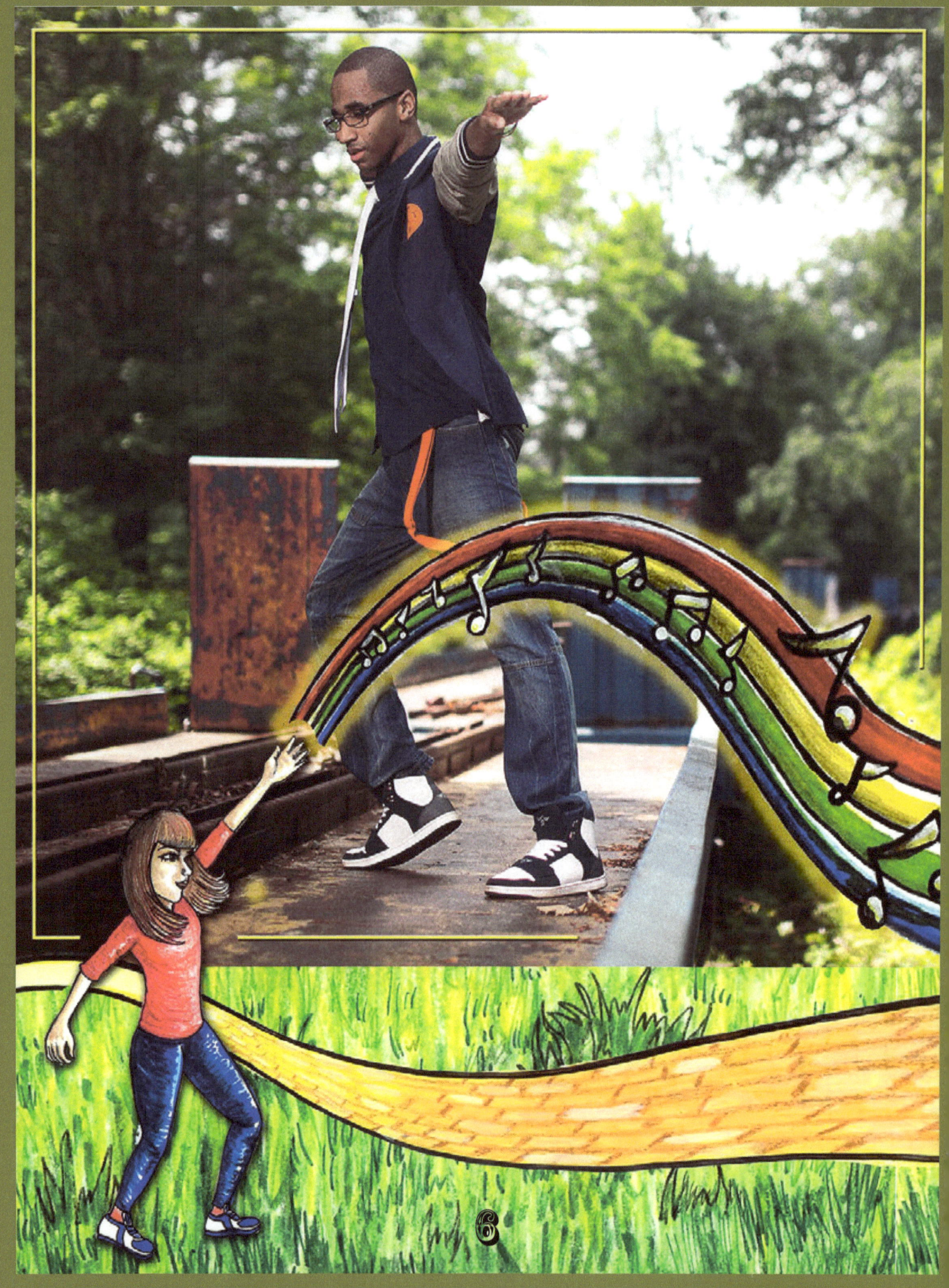

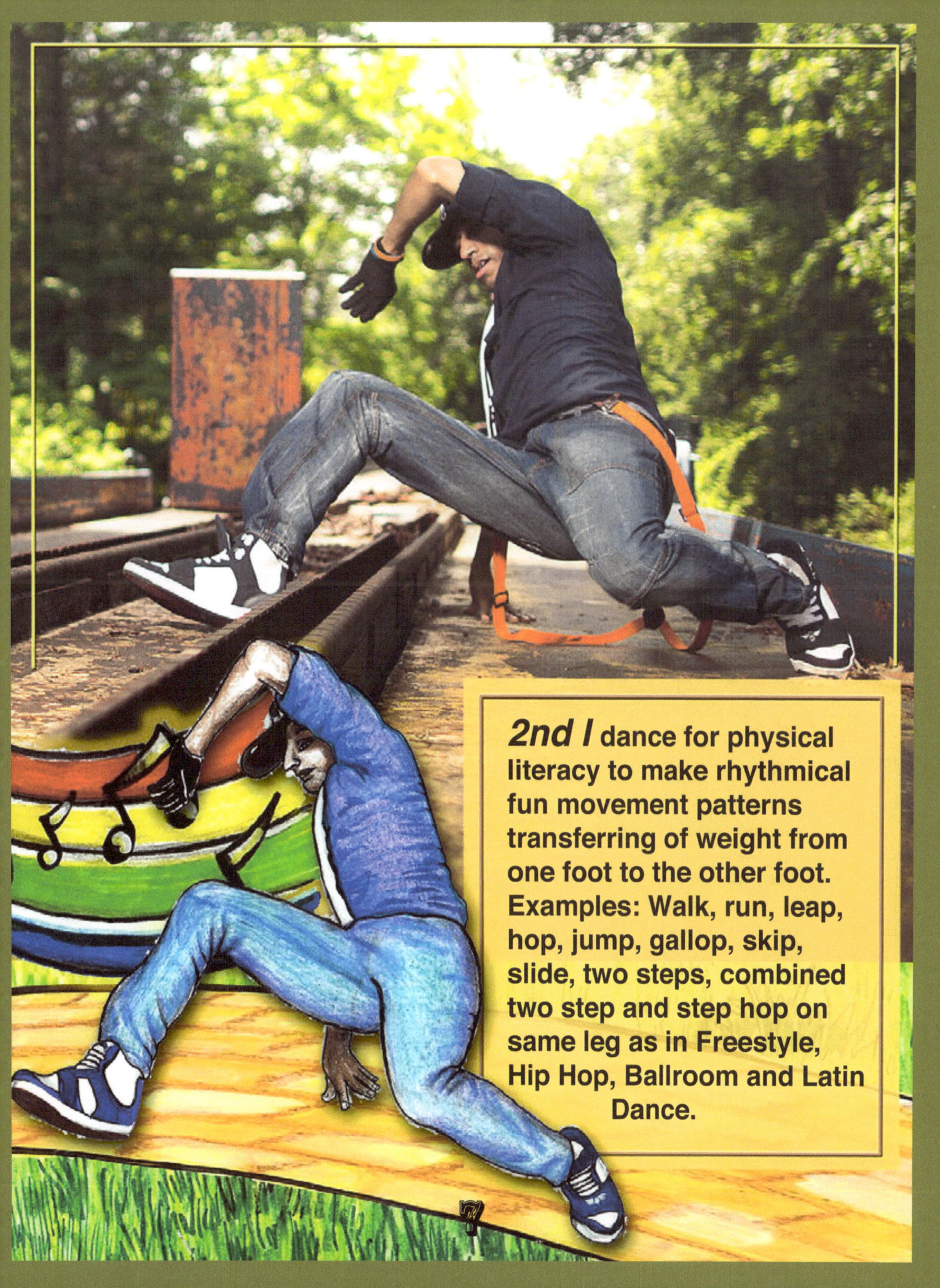

2nd I dance for physical literacy to make rhythmical fun movement patterns transferring of weight from one foot to the other foot. Examples: Walk, run, leap, hop, jump, gallop, skip, slide, two steps, combined two step and step hop on same leg as in Freestyle, Hip Hop, Ballroom and Latin Dance.

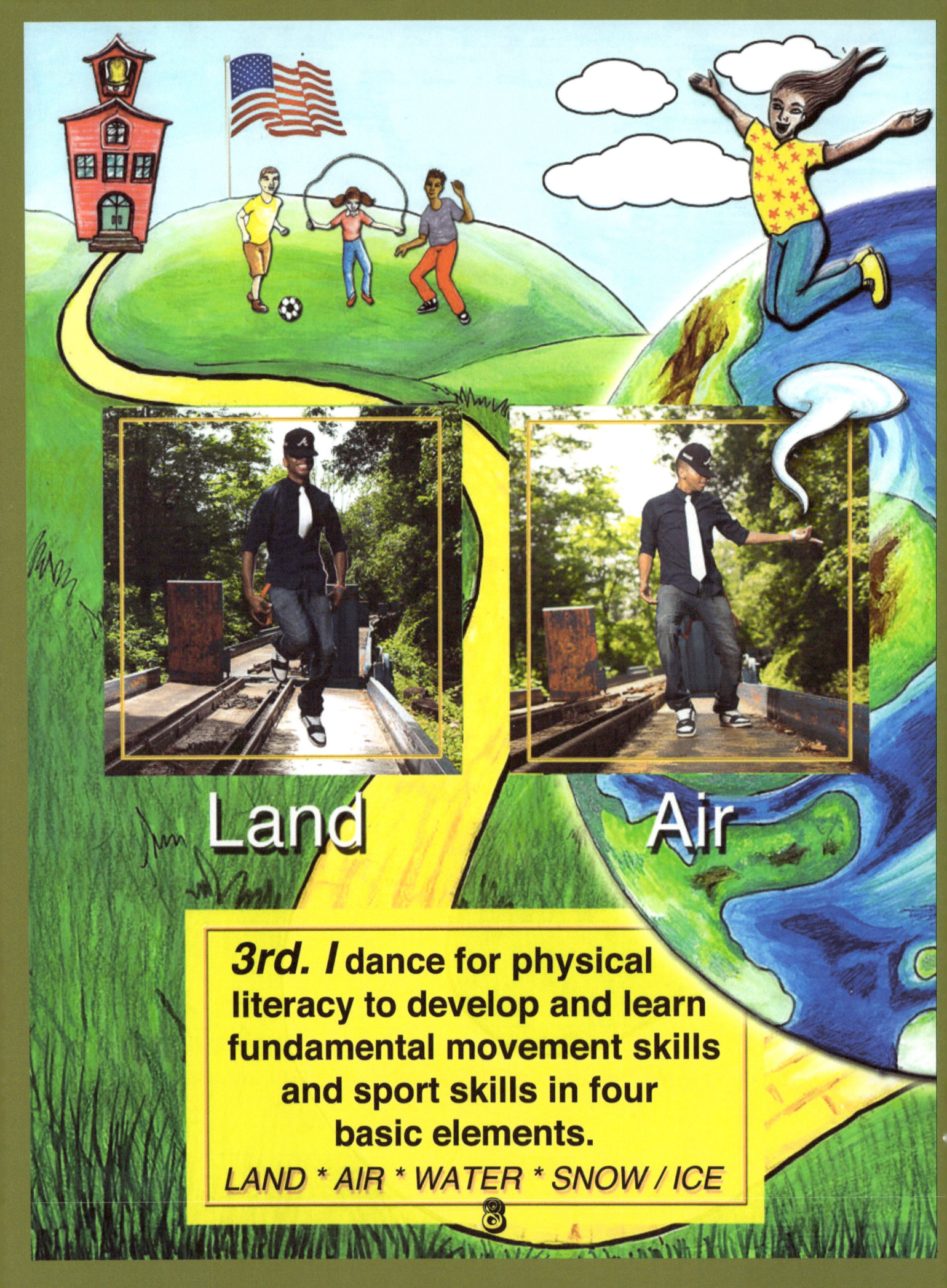

Land

Air

3rd. I dance for physical literacy to develop and learn fundamental movement skills and sport skills in four basic elements.

LAND * AIR * WATER * SNOW / ICE

8

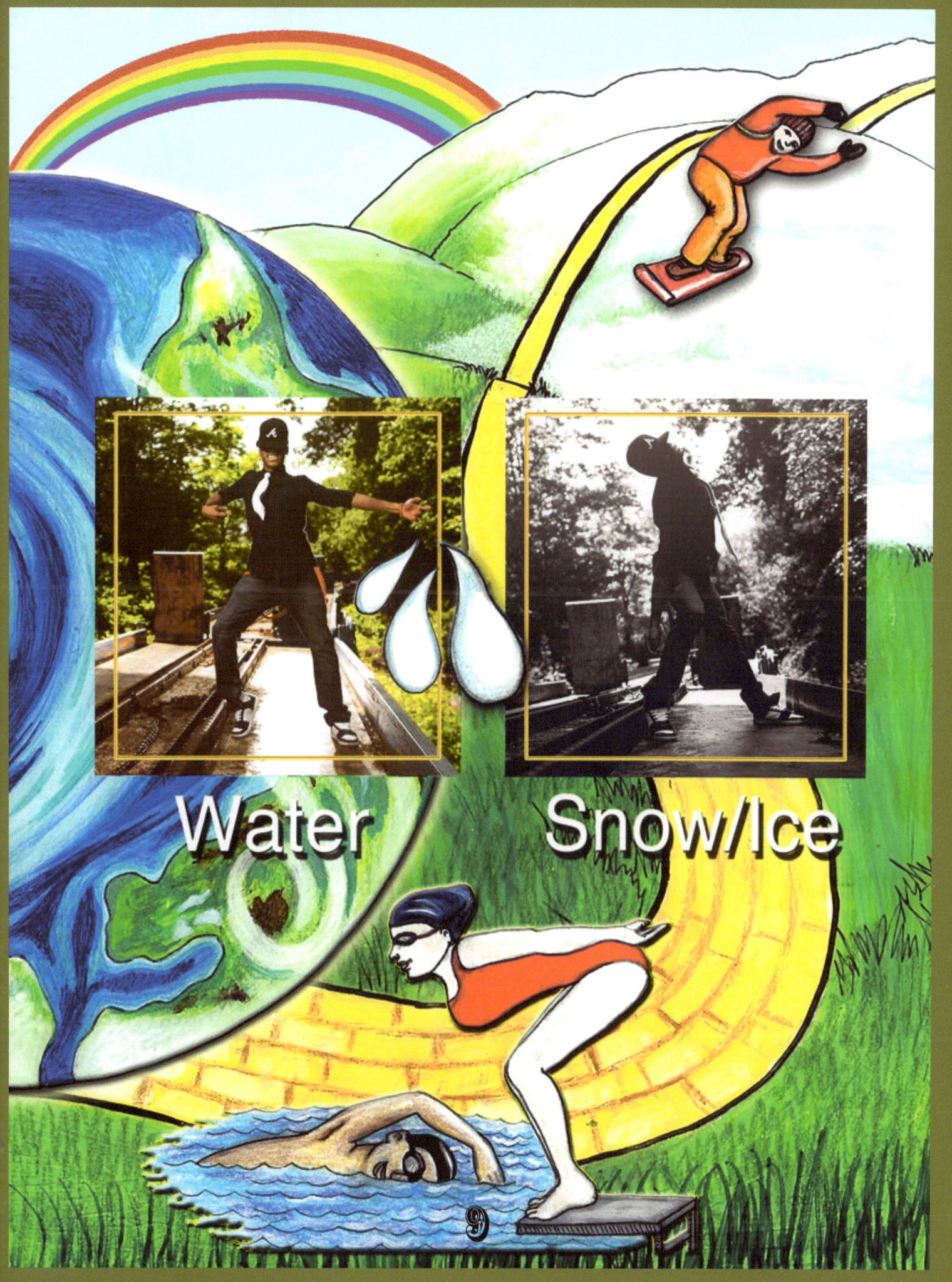

Water   Snow/Ice

9

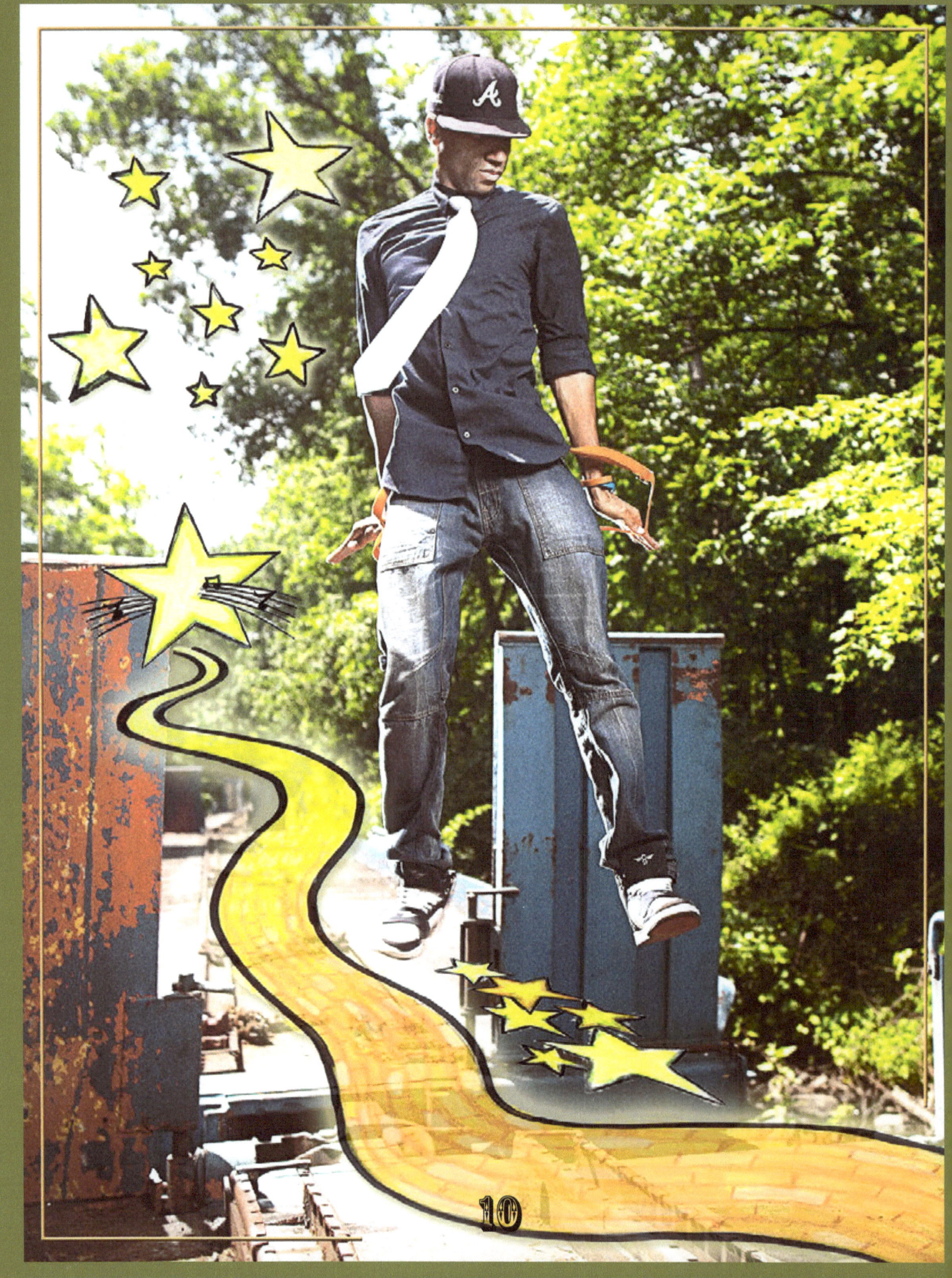

10

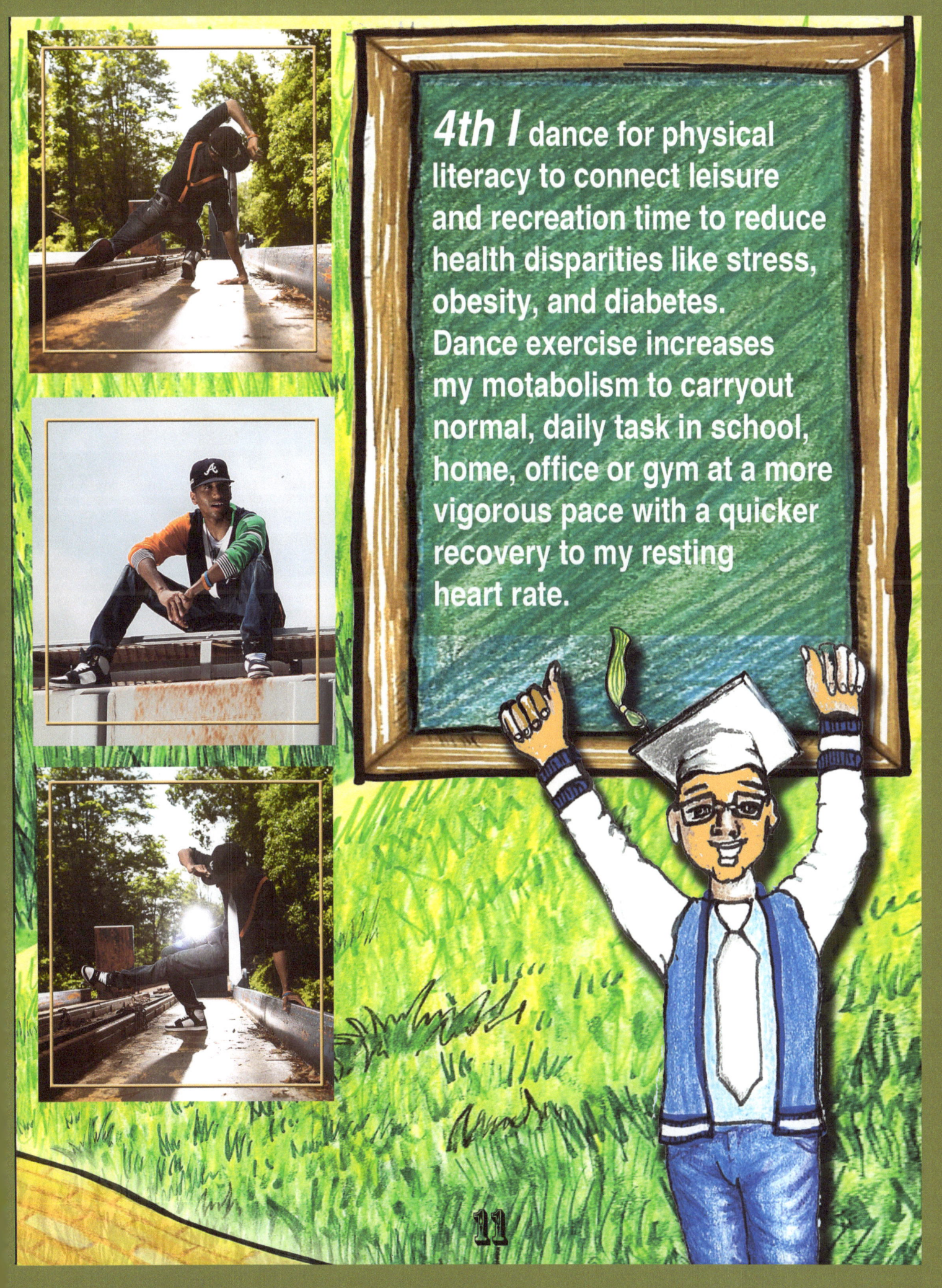

4th I dance for physical literacy to connect leisure and recreation time to reduce health disparities like stress, obesity, and diabetes. Dance exercise increases my motabolism to carryout normal, daily task in school, home, office or gym at a more vigorous pace with a quicker recovery to my resting heart rate.

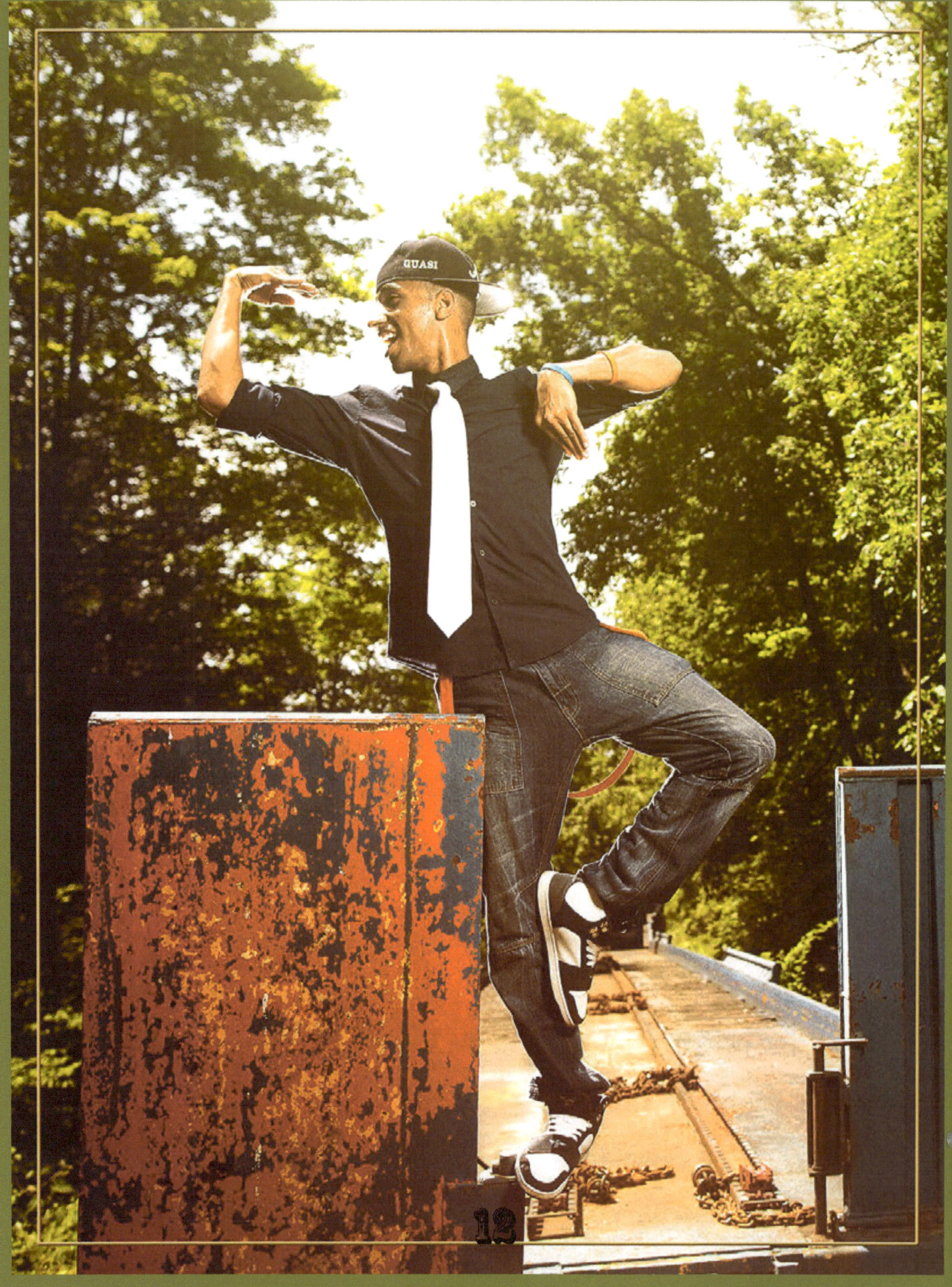

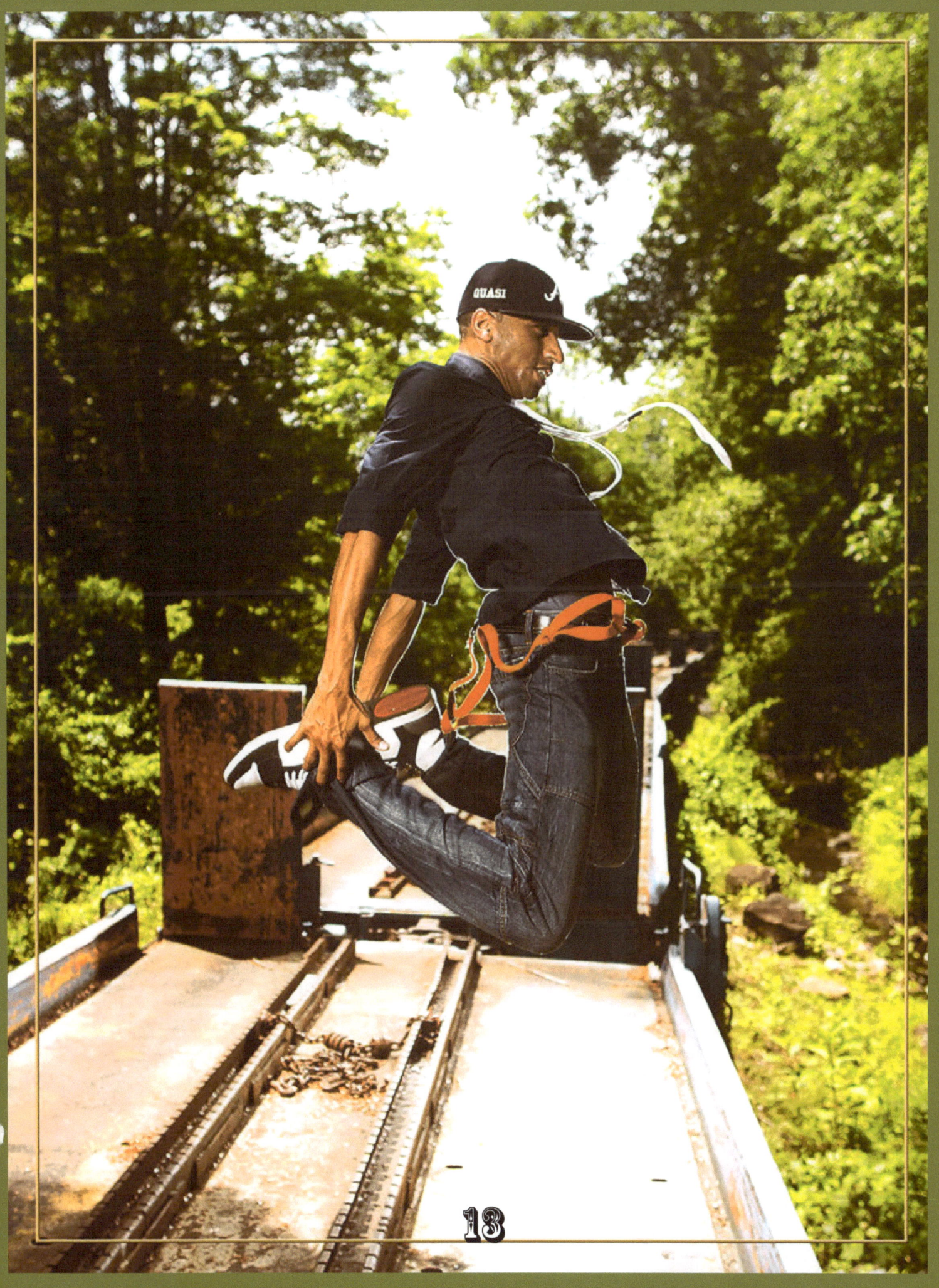

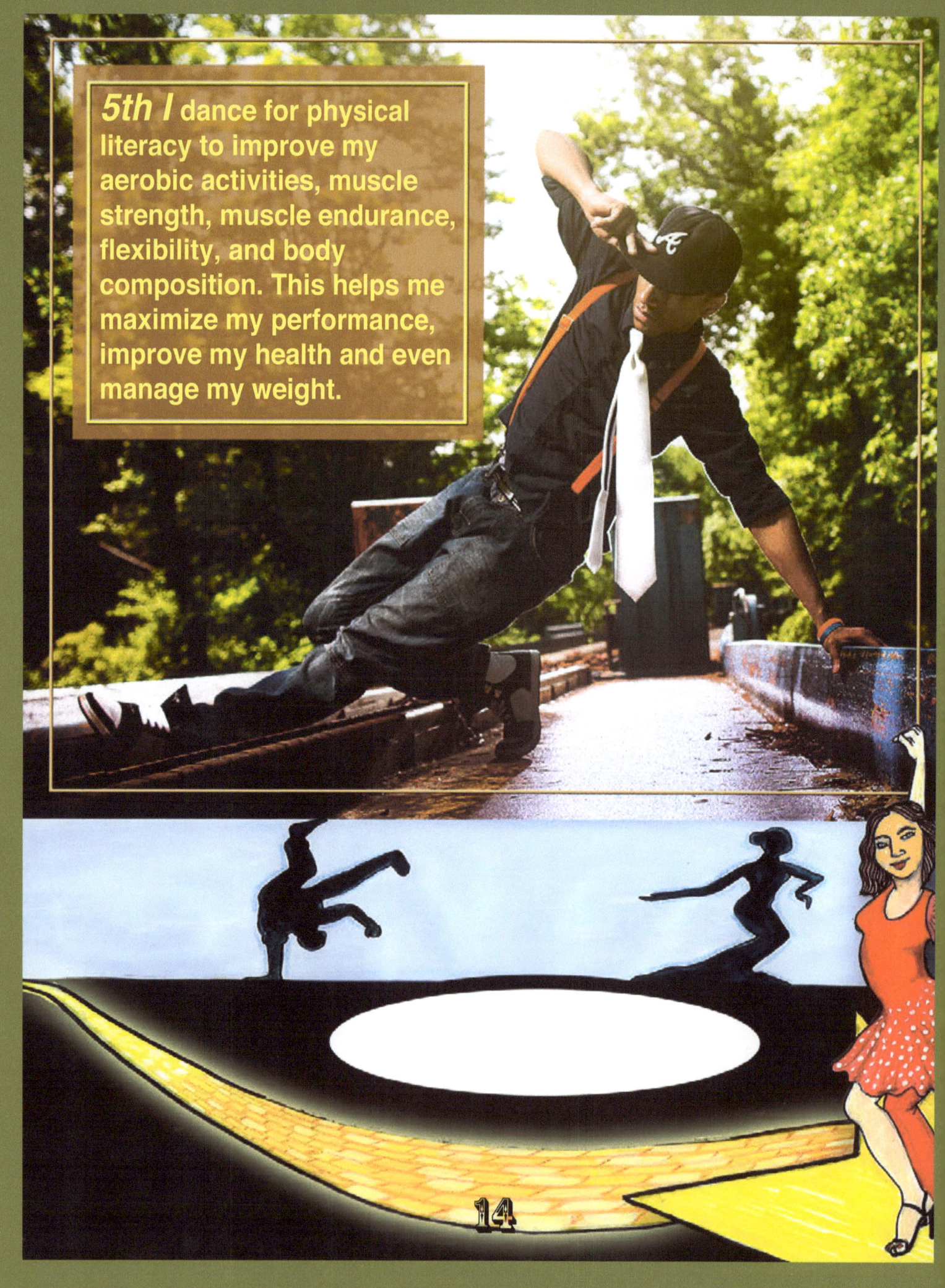

5th I dance for physical literacy to improve my aerobic activities, muscle strength, muscle endurance, flexibility, and body composition. This helps me maximize my performance, improve my health and even manage my weight.

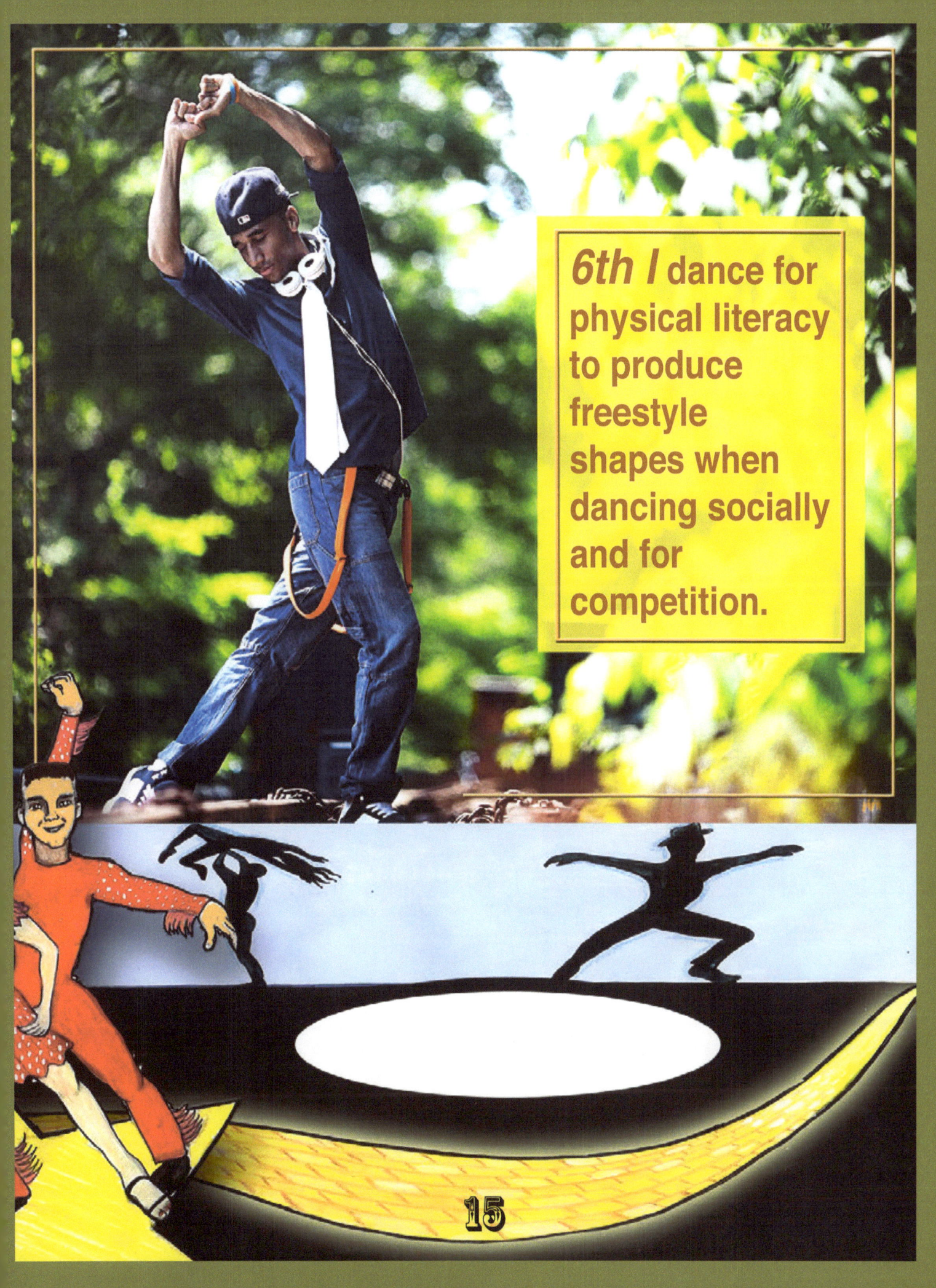

6th I dance for physical literacy to produce freestyle shapes when dancing socially and for competition.

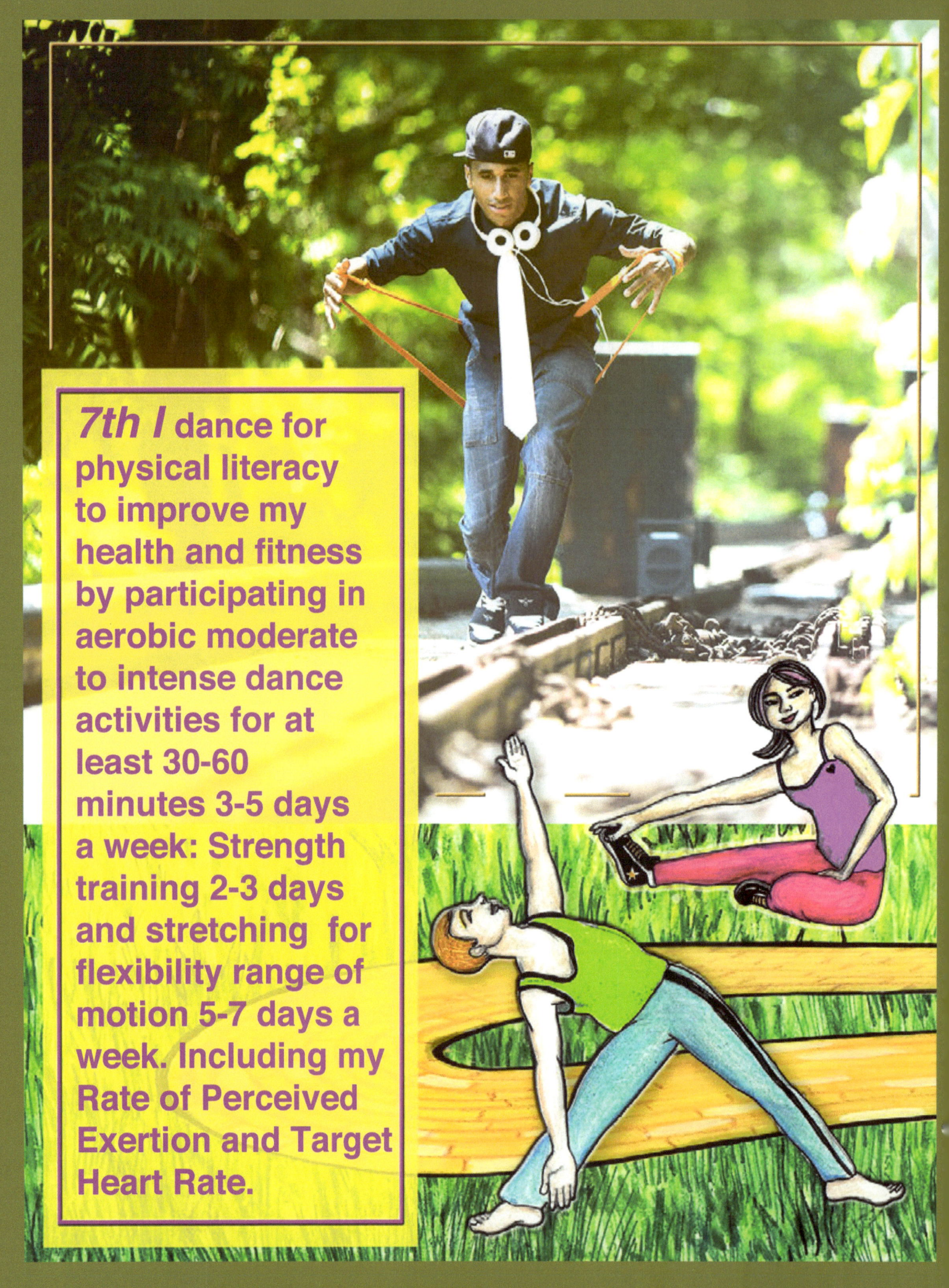

7th I dance for physical literacy to improve my health and fitness by participating in aerobic moderate to intense dance activities for at least 30-60 minutes 3-5 days a week: Strength training 2-3 days and stretching for flexibility range of motion 5-7 days a week. Including my Rate of Perceived Exertion and Target Heart Rate.

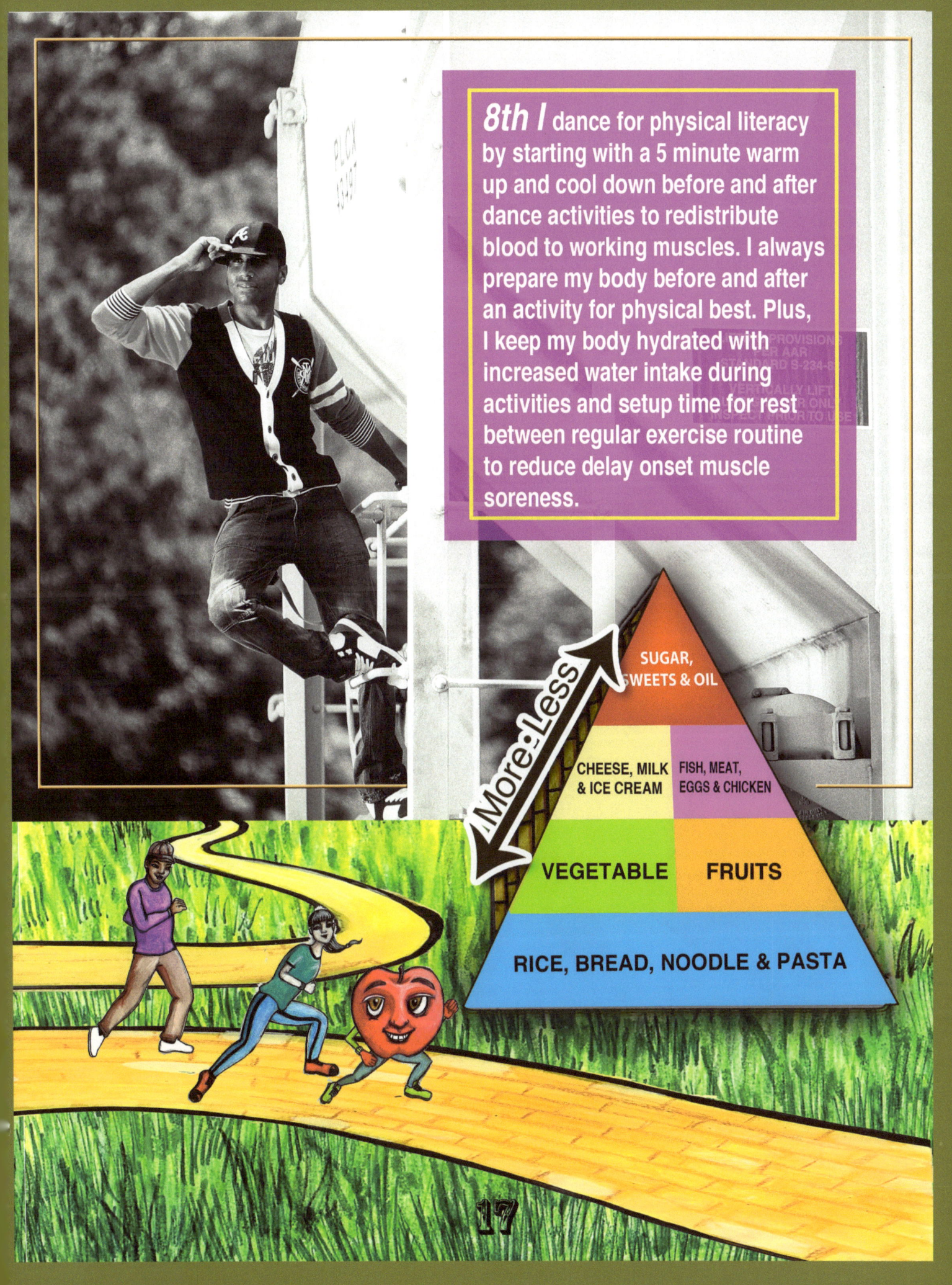

8th I dance for physical literacy by starting with a 5 minute warm up and cool down before and after dance activities to redistribute blood to working muscles. I always prepare my body before and after an activity for physical best. Plus, I keep my body hydrated with increased water intake during activities and setup time for rest between regular exercise routine to reduce delay onset muscle soreness.

More:Less

SUGAR, SWEETS & OIL

CHEESE, MILK & ICE CREAM

FISH, MEAT, EGGS & CHICKEN

VEGETABLE

FRUITS

RICE, BREAD, NOODLE & PASTA

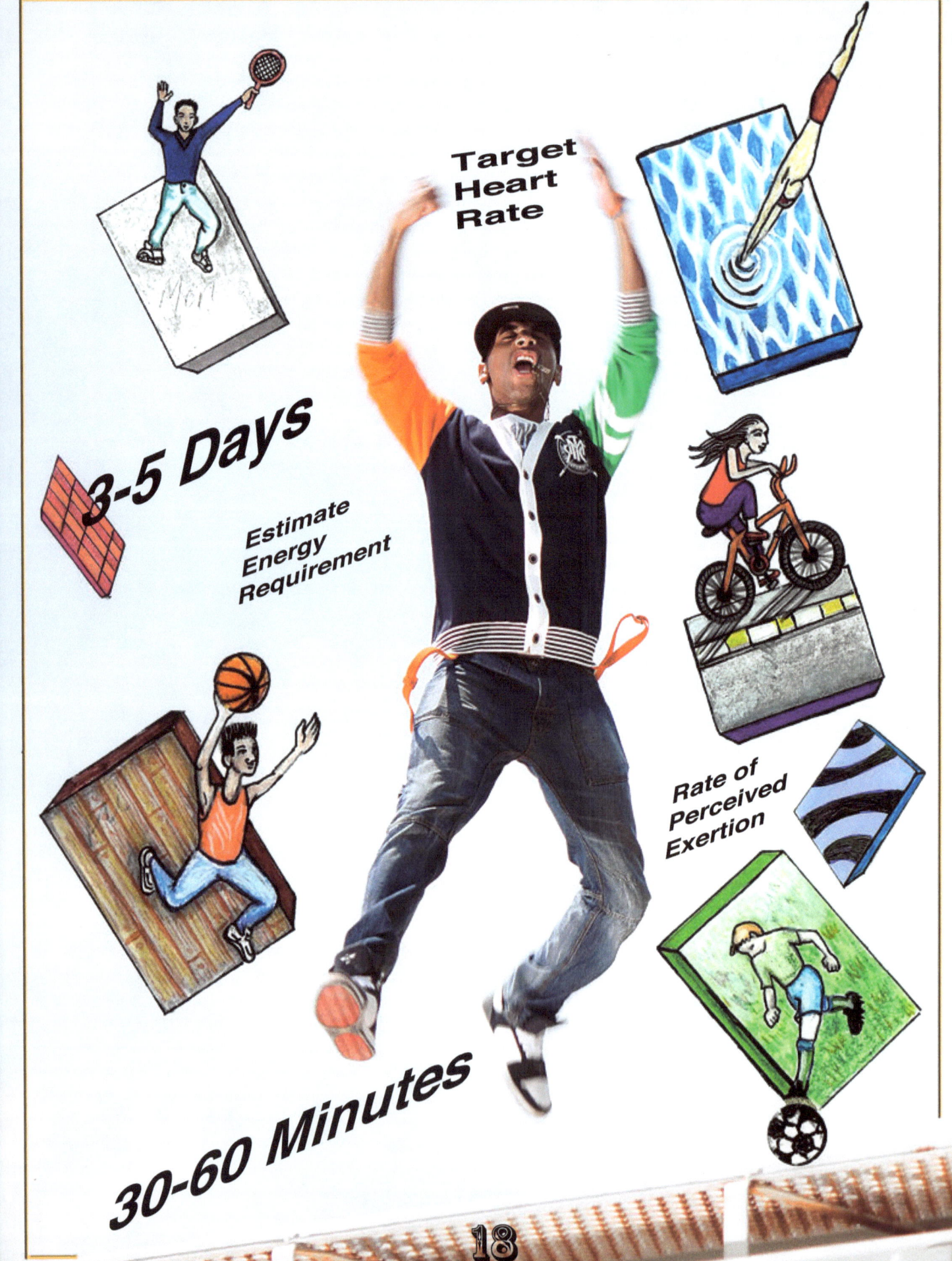

Target
Heart
Rate

3-5 Days

Estimate
Energy
Requirement

Rate of
Perceived
Exertion

30-60 Minutes

18

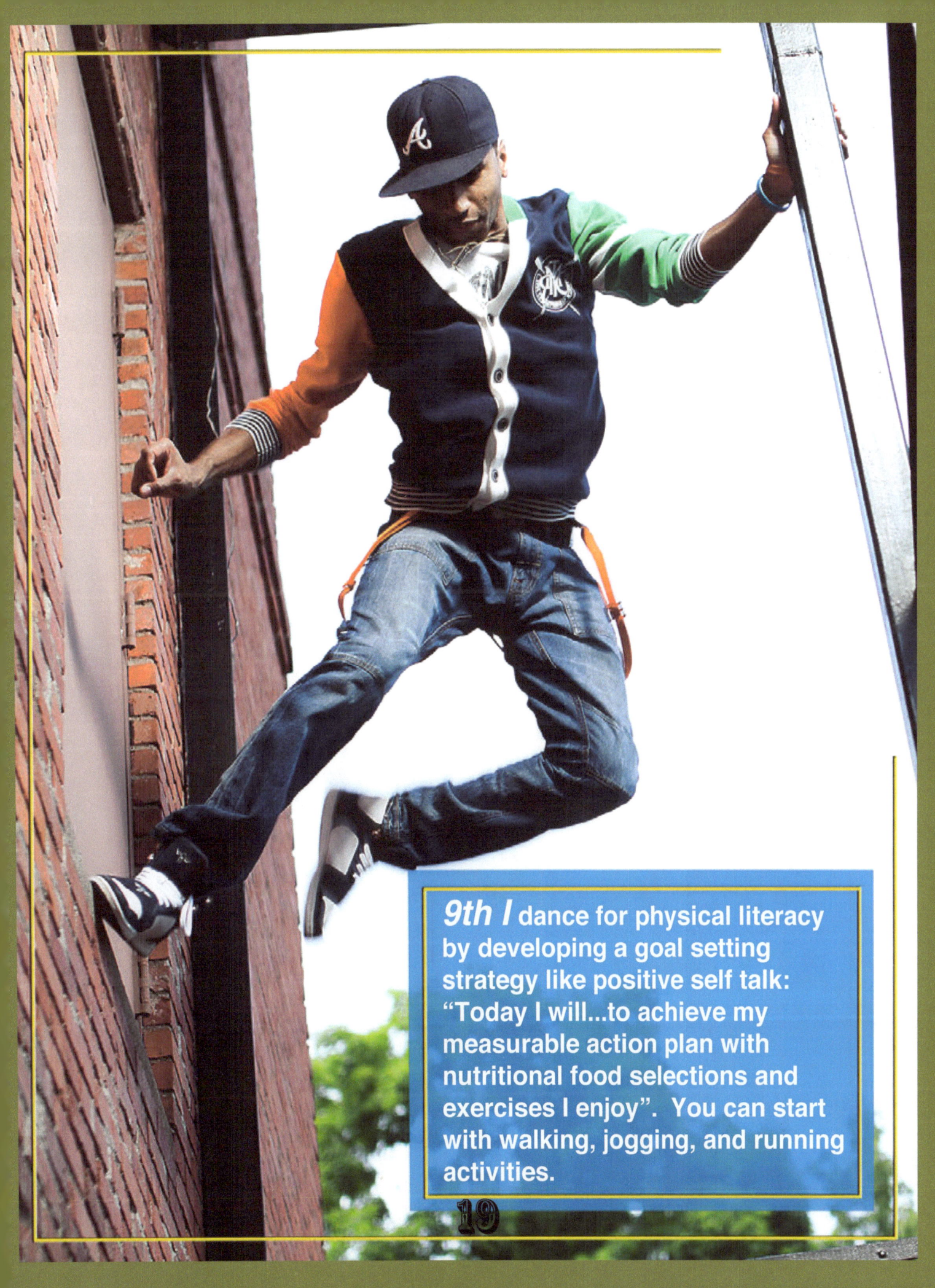

9th I dance for physical literacy by developing a goal setting strategy like positive self talk: "Today I will...to achieve my measurable action plan with nutritional food selections and exercises I enjoy". You can start with walking, jogging, and running activities.

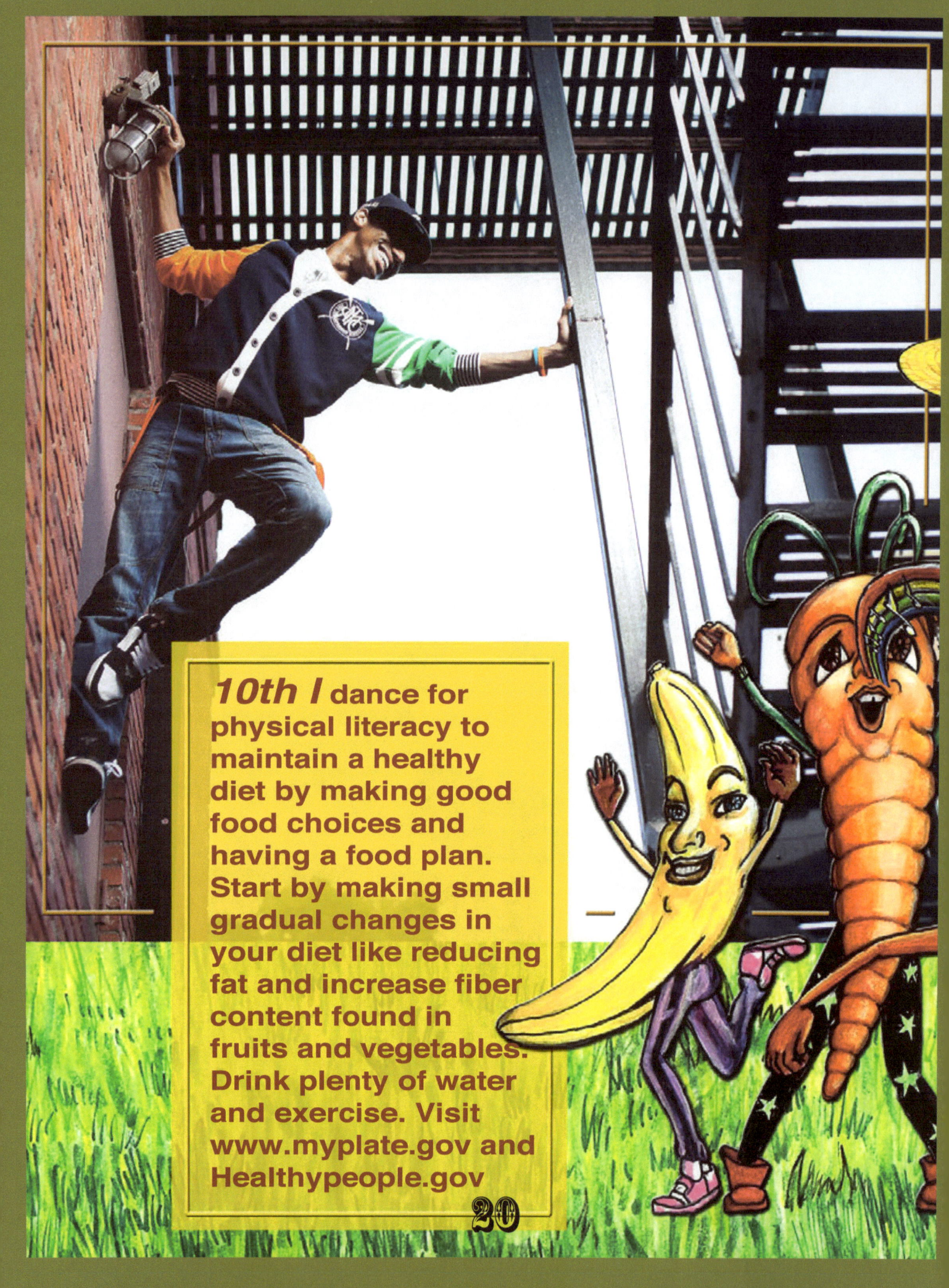

10th I dance for physical literacy to maintain a healthy diet by making good food choices and having a food plan. Start by making small gradual changes in your diet like reducing fat and increase fiber content found in fruits and vegetables. Drink plenty of water and exercise. Visit www.myplate.gov and Healthypeople.gov

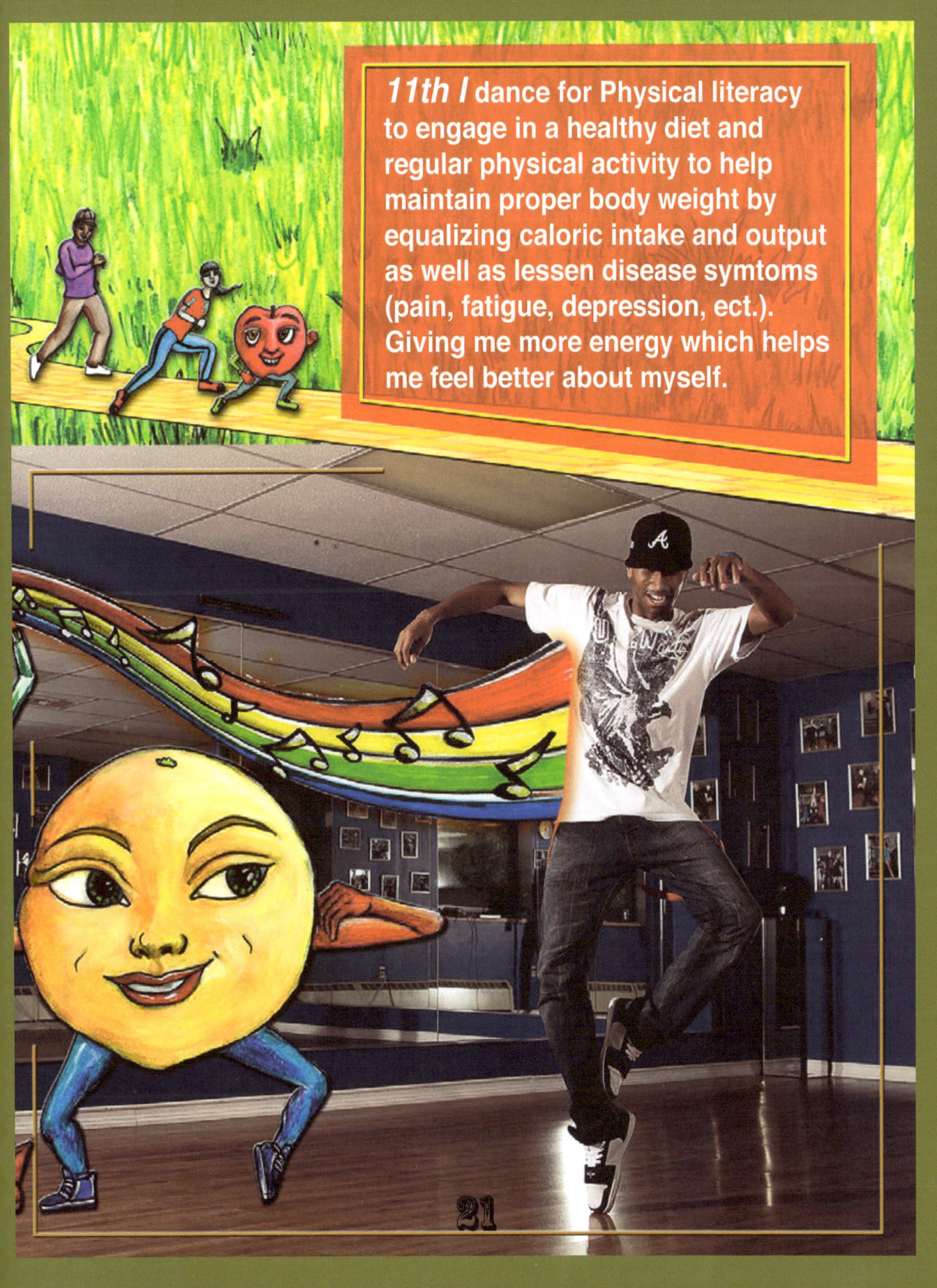

11th I dance for Physical literacy to engage in a healthy diet and regular physical activity to help maintain proper body weight by equalizing caloric intake and output as well as lessen disease symtoms (pain, fatigue, depression, ect.). Giving me more energy which helps me feel better about myself.

21

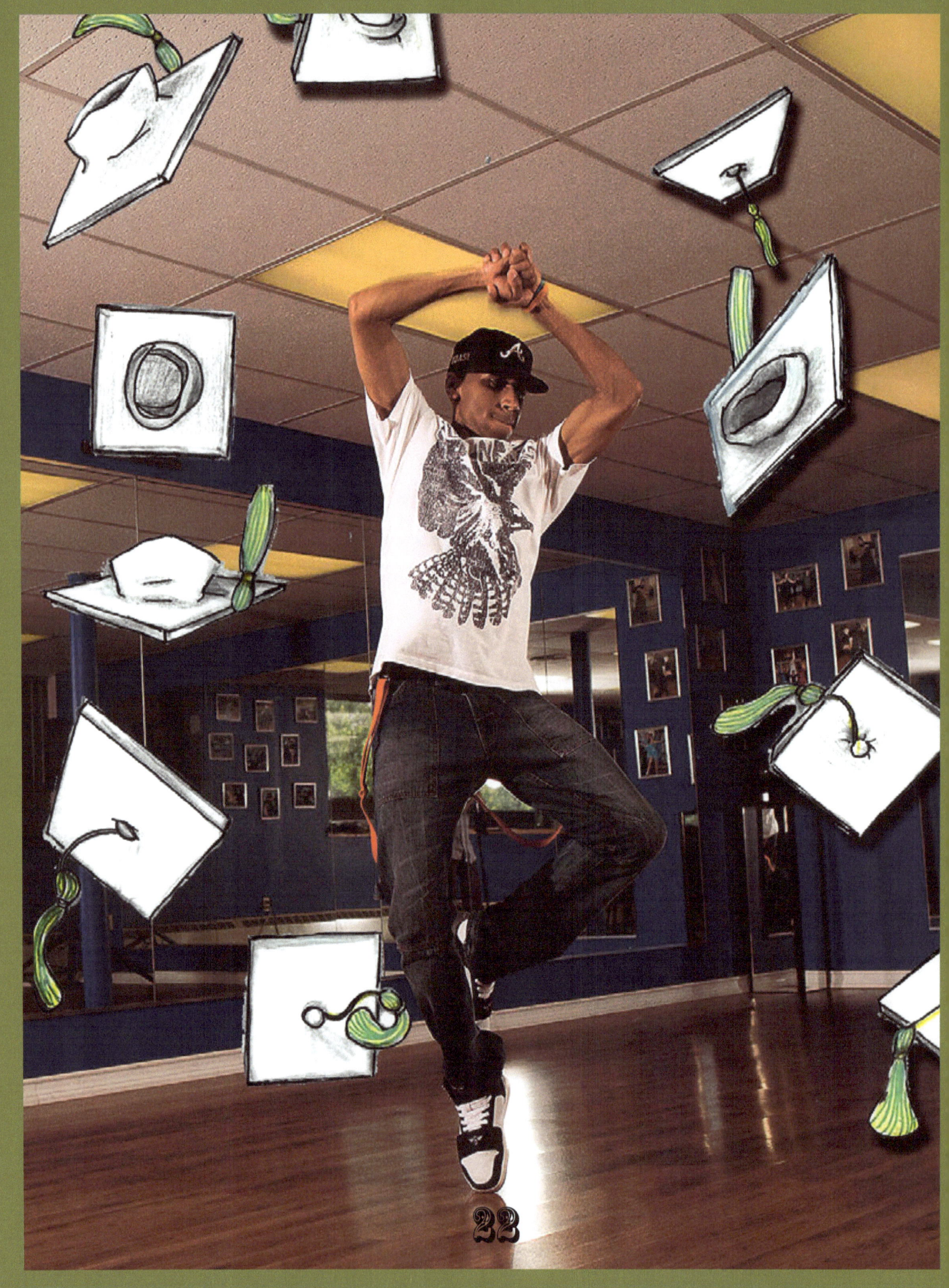

12th I dance for physical literacy promoting choices like dance to teach children, adolescents and adults to become physically literate (active across the four environments:
   LAND, AIR, WATER, SNOW / ICE
for leisure, recreation and sport.

Physical literacy is best achieved by combining health and fitness objectives. Start with a food plan and action plan to ensure your success by stating your goals and chosen exercise, time and place (environment) to exercise, and determine how long you will stick to a plan. For exercise activities 8-12 weeks is a reasonable time commitment for a new program. Join me as ambassadors of "I DANCE for PHYSICAL LITERACY 12 steps" Create your own pledge for staying active across your lifespan to maintain your physical best. To learn more consult with your community leaders, teachers, health professionals. Share your action plan with your family and friends. Become a lifelong learner.

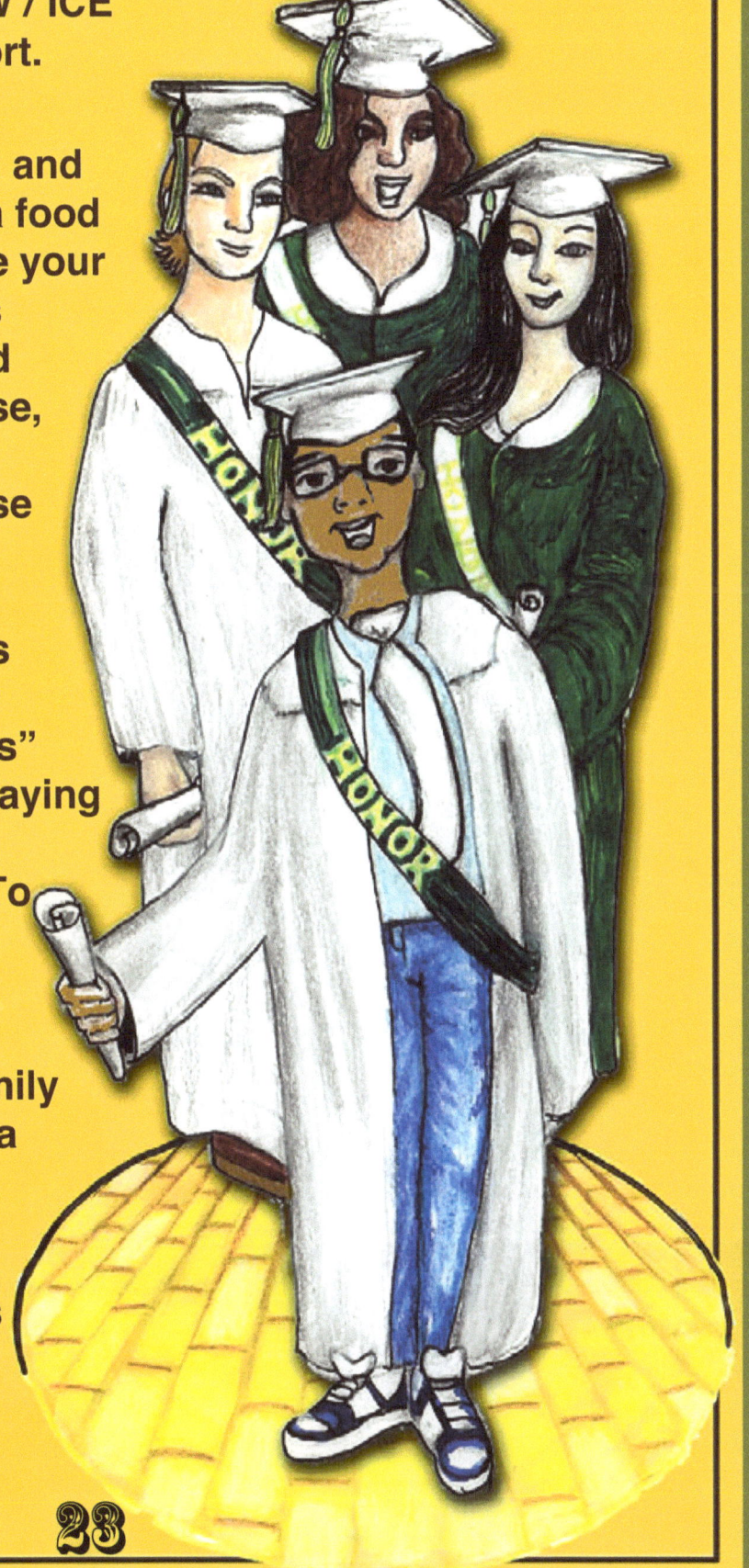

   Physical literacy helps sustain mental, physical and social well being at every fitness level.

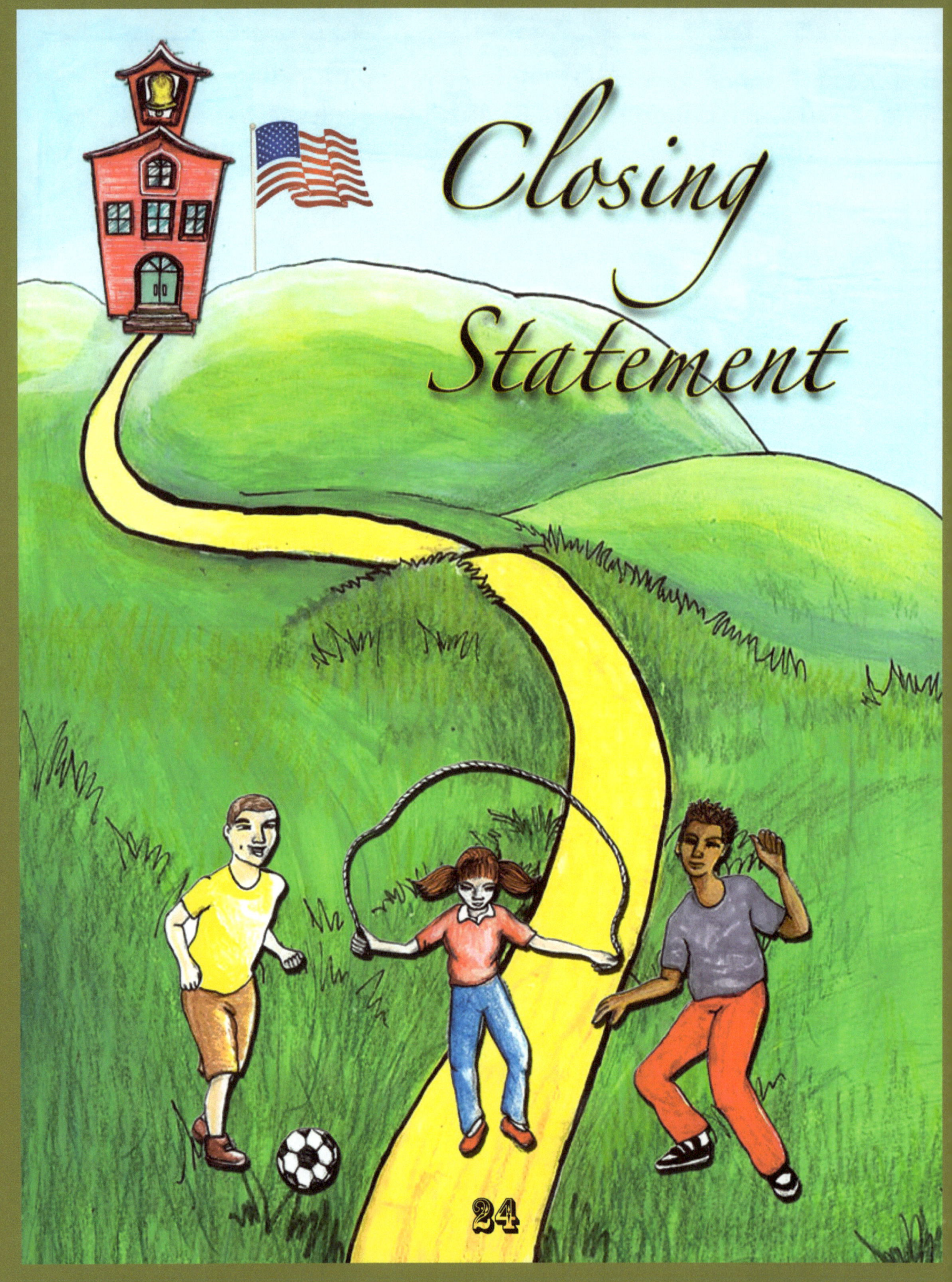

Closing Statement

24

*A*lthough dance is an ideal way to achieve a unique kind of physical education, it is not the only way to achieve physical literacy. Each individual is on a very unique journey towards developing physical literacy and could approach it in numerous ways. Whichever way you choose to approach your individual journey, ensure that it involves developing skills that will allow for a wide range of application and creative expression. This is the key to maintaining physical literacy: versatile application.

*M*any people may experience setbacks in developing physical literacy due to a range of physical limitations or circumstances, but do not let this discourage you. Find the right support or form a support team with a friend, teacher, instructor or health professional (Review The Wave article FORM A SUPPORT TEAM). With hard work, no setback will be too big to overcome. You can and will be physically literate. Remember the quality of your physical education is directly proportionate to the effort you are willing to put into it. The "I Dance for Physical Literacy 12 Steps" was created as an aspiring pledge and reflection to promote physical literacy and physical education ambassadorship. Providing a more comprehensive approach to health, fitness, leisure, recreation and sports by staying active in the four environments: Land, Air, Water, Snow and Ice as lifelong learners. Now turn the page using your favorate activity and complete the template for creating your personal Physical Literacy 12 step pledge. Display and share with your friends and family .

Steven C. McCartney IPO HSW MS

Physical Literacy 12 Step Total Fitness Chart

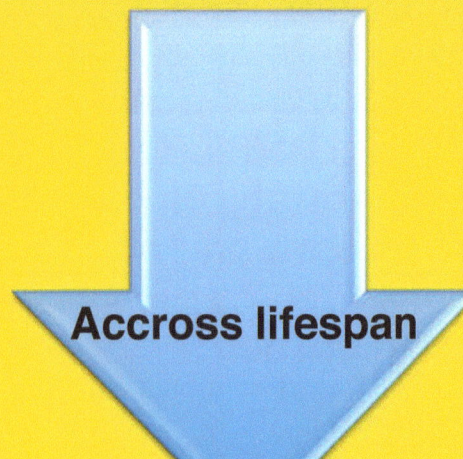

Accross lifespan

FITT Guidelines
Health-Related Components
Basic Training Principles
Skill-Related Components

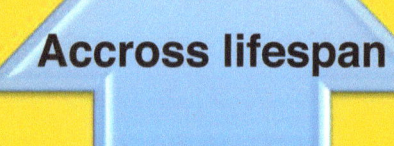

Physical Literacy 12 steps

Land

Air

Water

Snow / Ice

Accross lifespan

By Steven C. McCartney

FITT Guidelines	Health-Related Components	Basic Training Principles	Skill-Related Components
Frequency	Aerobic Fitness	Overload	Agility
Intensity	Muscular Strength	Progression	Balance
Time	Muscular Endurance	Specificity	Coordination
Type	Flexibility	Regularity	Power
	Body Composition	Individuality	Reaction
			Speed

Physical Literacy Ambassador: Longevity Quiz Assessment

Staying physically active is the single most effective way to ensure your physical, mental and social well-being (longevity). Participating in daily moderate exercise across your lifespan in activities you like can boost your Longevity Quotient. Now complete the six activity questions by selecting a letter then add up your score.

*Aerobic exercise involves repetitive submaximal contraction of major muscle groups, and requires oxygen for sustained muscle effort. Aerobic exercise are activities like walking, running, swimming and dancing.

** The 8 major muscle groups are chest, back, abdominals, biceps, triceps, shoulders, buttocks/hips, and legs.

Activity / Time	Select YOUR LQ POINTS		Maximum LQ Points	Your LQ Points
Weekly Aerobic * Exercise	a) 2 hours or more b) 1 to 2 hours c) 30 minutes s to 1 hour d) Less than 30 minutes per week	20 15 10 0	20	
Weekly Aerobic Exercise Level	a) Moderate or intense (e.g., brisk-walking 3-4 m/hr, 15-20 miles). b) Mix of moderate and light activity. c) Mostly light work-slow walking-gardening , house work. d) None	20 15 10 0	20	
Weight Training (lift weights, use weight machines, do resistance training)	a) Weight training for the 8 major-Muscle group** twice a week or more. b) Doing this once a week, or for a-few muscle groups only twice a week. c) Your daily job requires significant-Muscle exertion, but you don't do weight training. d) You do some weight training-weekly. e) You don't weight train regularly.	40 30 20 10 0	40	
Stretching and balance work (includes stretch exercises, yoga, tai chi, etc.)	a) You do some form of stretching -and/or balance work daily. b) You do this most of days / week. c) You do this some days/ weeks. d) You do this occasionally. e) You don't do any stretching/balancing.	10 8 5 3 0	10	
Warm up and Cool Down	a) You always warm up for at least-5 min. & cool down for 5 min. before and after exercise. b) You warm up and cool down often. c) You warm up and cool down some-times. d) You rarely warm up and cool down	5 4 3 0	5	
Form	a) You have received expert instruction-in weight training and stretching. b) You have received training in either-of these. c) You have read instructions about-These. d) You just plunged in without-instructions	5 3 2 0	5	
	TOTAL Longevity Quotient POINTS =			

Scores that equal:

91-100 = Physical Literacy 12 Steps Ambassadors! Maintain your activity stance across your lifespan and four environments.

81-90 = Congratulations! However review your action plan and problem solving techniques for Physical Literacy 12 Steps Ambassadors.

71-80 = You need to work out smarter so review, continue to learn and grow to stay physical literate.

Below 70 = Full fitness alert! This is a great opportunity to become a Physical Literacy 12 Step Ambassador and initiate an exercise plan as soon as possible. Remember consult with a health and fitness professional.

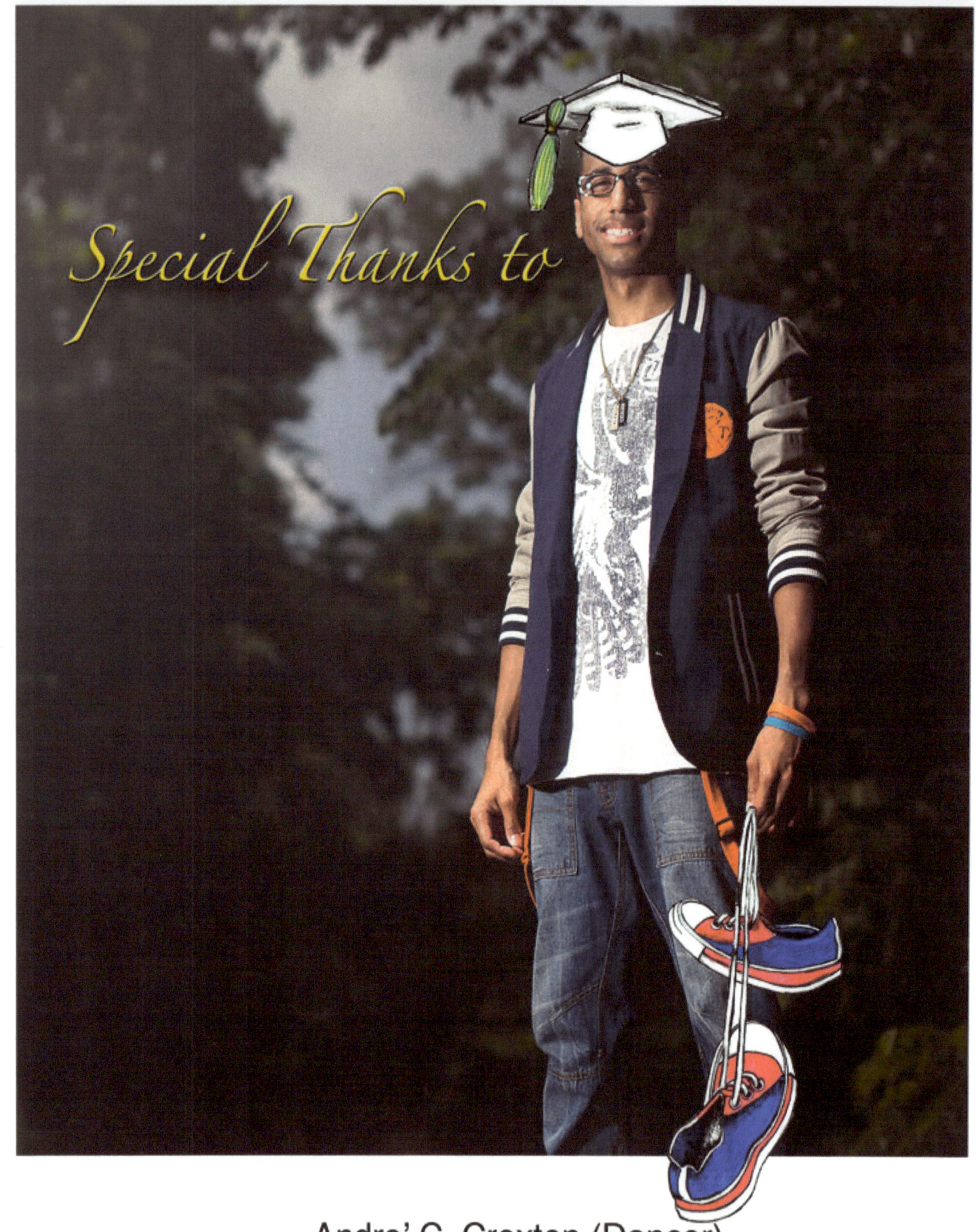

Special Thanks to

Andre' C. Croxton (Dancer)
Ainadel Ojeda (Illustrator)
Angelito Jusay (Photographer)

Physical Literacy Glossary

Aerobic energy – When the body is working (breathing) oxygen is used to help supply energy (ATP) to a person who is working.

Anaerobic energy – Process in which energy supplied without oxygen causing an oxygen debt. Creatine phosphate and glycolysis supply ATP when oxygen is not present for working muscles.

ATP- Adenosine triphosphate (ATP) is considered by biologists to be the "energy currency of life". It is the high-energy molecule that stores the energy we need to do just about everything we do. It is present in the cytoplasm and nucleoplasm of every cell, and essentially all the physiological mechanisms that require energy for operation obtain it directly from the stored ATP.

Ambassadorship – One who leads (representative) by diplomacy. Associated with leadership. Ex. Ambassador of good will.

Basic training principles – Consist of overload, progression, specificity, regularity, and individuality.

Blood pressure – Is the pressure of the blood within the arteries. It is produced primarily by the contraction of the heart muscle.

Body Composition – Relative percentage of fat and non fat tissue in the body.

Caloric Intake – The total number of calories in a daily diet allocation.

Calorie - A unit of heat used to indicate the amount of energy that foods will produce in the human body. plural cal·o·ries.

Cool down – A period following strenuous physical activity in which stretching or milder exercise is performed to allow the body gradually to return to normal redistribution of blood pooling.

Dance – To move one's feet or body, or both, rhythmically in a pattern of steps, especially to the accompaniment of music.

Depression – Is a mood disorder that causes a persistent feeling of sadness and loss of interest.

Diabetes – Diabetes mellitus refers to a group of diseases that affect how your body uses blood glucose, commonly called blood sugar. Glucose is vital to your health because it's an important source of energy for the cells that make up your muscles and tissues. It's also your brain's main source of fuel.

Diet – Food and drink considered in terms of its qualities, composition, and its effects on health. Visit www.myplate.gov

Estimate Energy Requirement – (EER) is the average dietary energy intake that is predicted to maintain energy balance in healthy, normal weight individuals of a defined age, gender, weight, height, and level of physical activity consistent with good health.

Exercise – A physical activity that is done in order to become stronger and healthier. : a particular movement or series of movements.

Exercise physiology – The scientific study of the acute and chronic metabolic responses of the human body to exercise, including biochemical and physiologic changes in the heart and skeletal muscles.

Fatigue – Reduction in the capacity of the neuromuscular system to carry out its functions as a result of physiological overwork and strain.

Fitness – Individual capability of the body of distributing inhaled oxygen to muscle tissue during increased physical effort.

FITT guidelines – Frequency, Intensity, Time, Type of activity Is a set of guidelines that help you set up a workout routine to fit your goals and fitness level while helping you get the most out of your exercise program. One of physical literacy components see chart.

Flexibility – The ability to move your body parts through their full range of motion without discomfort or pain.

Food Plan – A scheduled food intake recommendation that a person follows.

Food Pyramid – A food pyramid is defined as graphic representation of the food chain structure, which is used to show various forms predatory relationships. It can also be seen as a nutritional diagram that shows the principles of good nutrition. Fruits and vegetables are normally at the bottom of the pyramid which forms bulk of an healthy diet while fats and oils are found at the top. Visit www.myplate.gov

Free Style – Dance improvisation is not only about creating new movement but is also defined as freeing the body from habitual movement patterns.

Fruits – the sweet and fleshy product of a tree, bush or other plant that contains seed and can be eaten as food. Like blueberry, orang or apple.

Goal Setting – Motivational technique based on the concept that the practice of setting specific goals enhances performance, and that setting difficult goals results in higher performance than setting easier goals.

Heart Rate – The number of heartbeats per minute.

Health – Health is a state of complete physical, mental and social well-being and not merely the absence of disease or infirmity. WHO – World Health Organization.

Health Disparities – If a health outcome is seen in a greater or lesser extent between populations, there is disparity. Race or ethnicity, sex, sexual identity, age, disability, socioeconomic status, and geographic location all contribute to an individual's ability to achieve good health. Visit www.helathypeople.gov

Healthy Lifestyle – A healthy lifestyle is having the right amount of food and exercise, a way of life which must involve regular exercise where you, as a person, are in complete state of physical, social and mental well being, whilst having the ability to meet the demand of the environment without undue fatigue.

Health-related component – consist of five components: Aerobic fitness, muscular strength, muscular endurance, flexibility, and body composition.

Hydration - The process of providing an adequate amount of liquid to bodily tissues.

Leisure – Opportunity afforded by free time to do something of interest.

Life Long Learner – The ongoing, voluntary, and self-motivated pursuit of knowledge for either personal or professional reasons. Therefore, it not only enhances social inclusion, active citizenship, and personal development, but also self-sustainability, rather than competitiveness and employability.

Measurable outcome– Refer to data expressed as a number, percentage, or other quantifiable unit of measurement. A goal: What you hope to achieve and/or accomplish.

Movement Skills – Fundamental skills for movement are: static balance, sprint run, vertical jump, side gallop, catch, kick, hop, skip, leap, overarm throw, two-hand strike, and dodge.

Muscle Endurance – The ability of a muscle (slow twitch) to do continuous work over a long period of time

Muscle Strength – Muscular strength is the amount of force that muscles can exert against some form of resistance in a single effort. It is also known as physical strength. Strength is an important measure for fitness.

Muscle fiber – Muscle cells contain myofibrils that are composed of sarcomeres, uses chemical energy of ATP to generate tension, which, when greater than the resistance result in movement.

Obesity – A medical condition in which excess body fat has accumulated to the extent that it may have an adverse effect on health. Generally can be managed by diet and exercise.

Pain – A Physical suffering or discomfort caused by illness or injury.

Performance – The action or process of carrying out or accomplishing an action, task, or function.

Physical Fitness – A general state of health and well-being or specifically the ability to perform aspects of sports or occupations. Achieved through correct nutrition, exercise, hygiene and rest.

Physical Education – A systematic instruction in sports, exercises, and hygiene given as part of a school or college program.

Physical Literacy – Competence and confidence in a wide variety of physical activities in multiple environments (land, Air, Water, Ice/Snow) that benefit the healthy development of the whole person.

Pledge – A solemn promise or undertaking.

Recovery – A return to a normal state of health, mind, or strength.

Recreation – Something people do to relax or have fun: activities done for enjoyment.

Rest – A bodily state characterized by minimal functional and metabolic activities.

Resting Heart Rate – (RHR) refers to the number of times your heart beats in one minute while at rest. The average RHR is 70-80 beats per minute (BPM), though athletes may have resting heart rates as low as 40-50 BPM. RHR is often a measure of fitness -- as you become more fit, your RHR will decrease as your heart becomes more efficient.

Rate of Perceived Exertion– (RPE) The **RPE** scale is used to measure the intensity of your exercise. The **RPE** scale runs from 0 – 10 (easy – difficulty of an activity). Other types of RPE scales (Borg's) runs from 6 - 20.

Skill related components – Consist of agility, balance, coordination, power, reaction time, and speed.

Social Well Being – Social well-being is an end state in which basic human needs are met and people are able to coexist peacefully in communities with opportunities for advancement. This end state is characterized by equal access to and delivery of basic needs services (water, food, shelter, and health services), the provision of primary and secondary education, the return or resettlement of those displaced by violent conflict, and the restoration of social fabric and community life

Sportsmanship – Conduct (as fairness, respect for one's opponent, and graciousness in winning or losing) becoming to one participating in a sport.

Stress – A state of mental tension and worry or anxiety caused by problems in your life, work, etc.

Target Heart Rate – Heart rate range recommended for fitness workouts.

Total fitness – Consist of Fitness guidelines, health related components, Basic training principles, and skill related components within multiple environments (land, air, water, ice/snow)

Vegetables – Any plant whose fruit, seeds, roots, tubers, bulbs, stems, leaves, or flower parts are used as food, as the tomato, bean, beet, potato, onion, asparagus, spinach, or cauliflower.

Warm up – Activities should be preceded by warm-up activities. A proper warm up increase body and muscle temperature, increase blood flow, and may enhance performance. Generally 5-10 minutes before strenuous activity.

Weight Management – a long-term approach to a healthy lifestyle and total fitness. It includes a balance of healthy eating and physical exercise to equate energy expenditure (EER) and energy intake.

My Physical Literacy 12 Step Pledge

An aspiring pledge and reflection to physical literacy and physical education ambassadorship. Start first by reading this book. Then replace the word Dance with your favorite activities that you enjoy and make your Physical Literacy 12 step Pledge today.

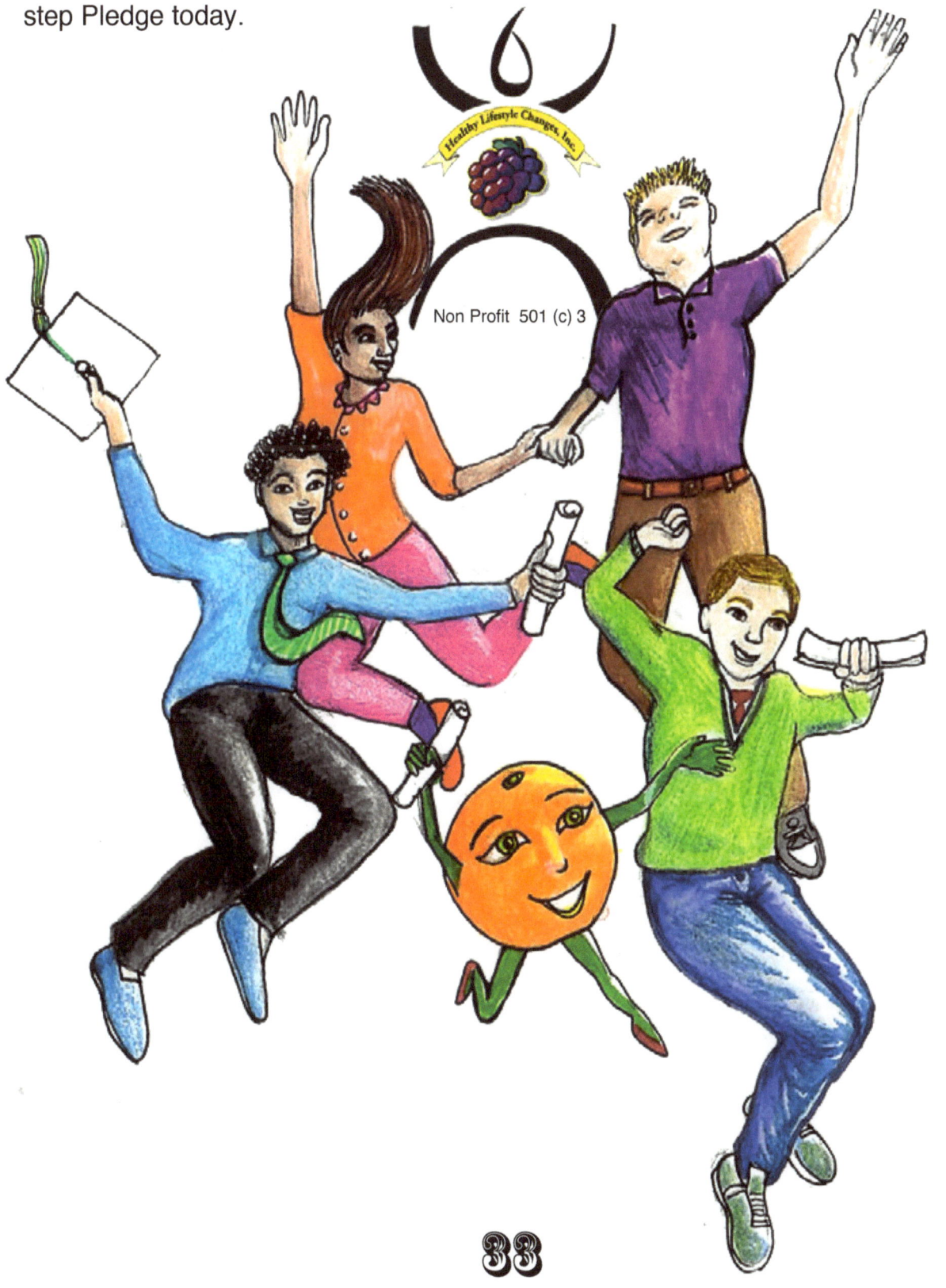

Non Profit 501 (c) 3

Physical Literacy
12 Step Pledge
Certificate

My Physical Literacy 12 Step Pledge

1st I _____ for physical literacy to keeps my body healthy and physically fit. When I stay physically active it helps keep me mentally, physically and socially connected with lifelong learning and Healthy Lifestyle Changes. I dance as a cultural activity that reveal the rich and varied forms of simple or complex movements that interconnect aspects of body, space and effort.

2nd I _____ for physical literacy to make rhythmical fun movement patterns transferring of weight from one foot to the other foot. Examples: Walk, run, leap, hop, jump, gallop, skip, slide, two steps, combined two-step and step hop on same leg as in _____, _____ and _____.

3rd I _____ for physical literacy to develop and learn fundamental movement skills and sport skills in four basic elements: LAND, AIR, WATER, and SNOW/ICE.

4th I _____ for physical literacy to connect my leisure and recreation time to reduce health disparities like stress, obesity, and diabetes. Dance exercise increases my motabolism to carryout normal, daily task in school, home, office or gym at a more vigorous pace with quicker recovery to my resting heart rate.

5th I _____ for physical literacy to improve my aerobic activities, muscle strength, muscle endurance, flexibility and body composition. This helps me maximize my performance, improve my fitness and even manage my weight.

6th I _____ for physical literacy to produce freestyle shapes and when _____ socially and for competition.

7th I _____ for physical literacy to improve my health and fitness by participating in aerobic moderate to intense dance activities for at least 45-60 minutes 3-5 days; Strength training 2-3 days; and stretch for flexibility range of motion 5-7 days a week. This should include my rate of perceived exertion and Target Heart Rate.

8th I _____ for physical literacy by starting with 5 min warm up and cool down before and after _____ _____activities to redistribute blood to working muscles. I always prepare my body before and after an activity for physical best. Plus I keep my body hydrated with increased water intake during activities and setup time for rest between regular exercise routine to reduce delay onset muscle soreness.

9th I _____ for physical literacy by developing a goal setting strategy like positive self-talk "Today I will … to achieve my measurable action plan with goals and chosen exercises I enjoy". You can start with walking, jogging, and running activities.

10th I _____ for physical literacy to maintain a healthy diet by making good food choices and having a food plan. Start by making small gradual changes in your diet like reducing fat and increase fiber content found in fruits and vegetables drink plenty of water and exercise. Learn more at www.myplate.gov and www.healthypeople.gov.

11th I _____ for physical literacy to engage in a healthy diet and regular physical activity to help maintain proper body weight by equalizing caloric intake and output as well as lessen disease symptoms (pain, fatigue, depression, etc.). Giving you more energy, and help you feel better about yourself.

12th I _____ for physical literacy promoting choices like _____ to teach children, adolescents and adults to become physically literate (active across the four environments: Land, air, water, snow/ice) for leisure, recreation and sport. Physical literacy is best achieved by combining health and fitness objectives. Start with food plan and action plan to ensure your success by stating your goals and chosen exercise, time and place (environment) to exercise, how long you will stick to plan. For exercise activities 8-12 weeks is a reasonable time commitment for a new program.

I Pledge to Physical Literacy 12 Step described above. I will use strategies and rewards to achieve the goals that will contribute to Physical Literacy 12 Step Pledge and physical education ambassadorship.

Signed_____

Witness: _____

Non Profit 501(c) 3

www.ingramcontent.com/pod-product-compliance
Lightning Source LLC
Chambersburg PA
CBHW041530280526
45792CB00004B/1446